Respiratory Pharmacology and Toxicology

Mannfred A. Hollinger, Ph.D.

Associate Professor of Pharmacology
Department of Pharmacology
School of Medicine
University of California
Davis, California

D1713943

A Volume in the Series
SAUNDERS MONOGRAPHS IN
PHARMACOLOGY AND THERAPEUTICS

Consulting Editor
Ronald J. Tallarida, Ph.D.

1985
W. B. SAUNDERS COMPANY
PHILADELPHIA   LONDON   TORONTO   MEXICO CITY
RIO DE JANEIRO   SYDNEY   TOKYO   HONG KONG

W. B. Saunders Company: West Washington Square
                         Philadelphia, PA 19105

Library of Congress Cataloging in Publication Data

Hollinger, Mannfred A.
Respiratory pharmacology and toxicology.

(Saunders monographs in pharmacology and therapeutics)
1. Respiratory agents—Physiological effect.   2. Respiratory
   organs—Effect of drugs on.   3. Respiratory therapy.
   4. Respiratory organs—Diseases—Chemotherapy.
   I. Title.   II. Series. [DNLM: 1. Respiratory System—drug
   effects.   2. Respiratory Tract Diseases—drug therapy.
   WF 145 H741r]

RM388.H65 1985   615'.72   84–27621

ISBN 0–7216–1617–8

Respiratory Pharmacology and Toxicology   ISBN   0–7216–1617–8

Last digit is the print number: 9   8   7   6   5   4   3   2   1

This book is dedicated to those people who have played significant roles in my life. To my parents I express my gratitude for providing direction and unending support in important ways. I thank my wife, Georgia, for the contributions she has made and for the encouragement she has given me. My sons, Randy and Chris, in their own ways, have inspired me to accept my challenges as they do in their lives. I also acknowledge the other special friends who, in various ways, have made important positive contributions to my life.

Preface

The fields of respiratory toxicology and pharmacology have developed independently over the years. Today, information relating to these areas can be obtained from many widely divergent sources. This book aims to assemble, condense and, when possible, integrate important fundamental aspects of these subjects to describe the respiratory system. Development of this text has been guided by the desire to be economical in topic selection and concise in presentation to provide an overview of important areas, and to facilitate the reader's task of becoming acquainted (or reacquainted) with the respiratory system.

Historically, the respiratory process of the lung has received the most study, and there is now a reasonably good detailed understanding of the physiology, mechanics, neurology, and physical chemistry of breathing. In recent years, however, more and more research efforts have been focused on the lung to understand how it functions as a target organ for both toxicants and drugs, as well as to delineate its nonrespiratory functions. Interest in the lung has therefore been extended from the physiologist to the pharmacologist and toxicologist. Clinical interest in these perspectives has also increased as more lung injury is now occurring as a result of exposure to toxic environmental chemicals, as well as of side effects from drugs.

Attempting to combine both pharmacologic and toxicologic aspects of the respiratory system in a single monograph has a logical basis, for several reasons. First, because the principles of pharmacology and toxicology are essentially interchangeable, coordinated coverage is reasonably straightforward and appropriate principles are mutually applicable. Aureolus Paracelsus (1493–1541), the grandfather of pharmacology, observed that "It is only the dose which makes a thing a poison." Although he was not technically correct, the thrust of the observation is, nevertheless, germane. Second, by dealing with both fields, it is hoped that important principles will be reinforced. For example, factors such as dose, exposure time, physical state, and rate of elimination are equally important in regulating the dynamics of both toxin and drug within the respiratory system.

Chapter 1 describes the basic anatomy of the respiratory system, with the morphology of the various regions being presented, as well as

iv

important properties of the component cells, vascular system, and nerve supply. Chapter 2 reviews the essential features of ventilation and oxygen transport; the effects of drugs and toxins on hemoglobin binding of oxygen are described, as are the effects of drugs that alter ventilation either centrally or peripherally, and directly or indirectly. Chapter 3 deals with nonrespiratory functions of the lung, with consideration of basic amine accumulation, activation and inactivation of endogenous substances, and xenobiotic metabolism; the process of metabolic activation of toxins and its role as a mechanism in lung injury are also introduced. Chapter 4 discusses asthma and its treatment, and the relative advantages and disadvantages of the major antiasthmatic drugs are presented. Chapter 5 emphasizes the lung as a route of drug administration; inhalational drugs such as oxygen and general anesthetics are discussed, with a review of principles governing their actions.

The most common ailments affecting the respiratory system are the common cold and other viral infections. Drugs used for the self-medication of upper respiratory tract infections are discussed in Chapter 6, with particular emphasis on decongestants and antitussives, and a critical assessment of antihistamines. Chapter 7 deals with hay fever, the most common allergic response of the respiratory tract. Its underlying immunologic process is described, especially the role of histamine and antihistamines, and the role of allergy in the development of asthmatic episodes is also considered. Chapter 8 discusses miscellaneous drugs used in respiratory therapy, such as mucokinetic agents, diagnostic radionuclides, and drugs used to treat pulmonary embolism. Chapter 9 analyzes how the lung responds to injury, with particular emphasis on reflexes, mucous secretion, and macrophages; variable sensitivity and patterns of cell renewal, and the components and temporal relationship of inflammation and tissue repair are also considered. Chapter 10 describes various types and sources of external respiratory hazards: major environmental, occupational, clinical, and abused substances are considered on the basis of their relationship to the respiratory system.

Decisions relating to the selection and organization of the material in this book were predicated on my subjective considerations. My predominating concern was to provide an updated and concise overview that would be valuable to clinicians, researchers, and students who desire either a reasonably quick review of the subject or a brief introduction. This book should, therefore, prove useful to a wide range of readers, including pulmonologists and undergraduate and graduate students, as well as nursing and medical students. I would welcome suggestions and advice from readers to strengthen and improve future editions.

Contents

Basic Lung Structure and Function

PRINCIPAL ARCHITECTURAL COMPONENTS OF THE RESPIRATORY SYSTEM

The basic structure of the adult human respiratory system consists of a series of bifurcating ventilatory conduits of varying length, flexibility, and diameter, which terminate in thin-walled sacs. These branches connect the external atmosphere with the internal vasculature, and are composed of conducting airways (trachea, bronchi, and bronchioles), transitory ducts, and respiratory zones (alveoli) (Fig. 1–1). Each has characteristic features and functions that are not only important to normal physiology but that also significantly influence toxin and drug disposition and dynamics.

Examination of the human respiratory "tree" reveals that it is a structure of considerable asymmetry. Most humans, for example, have three lobes on their right lung and generally two lobes on their left. Furthermore, the right main stem bronchus angles off at 20 to 30° from the midline, whereas the left angles off more acutely at 45 to 55°. It has been determined that it is possible to reach the alveoli from the trachea by traversing as few as eight branches or as many as twenty or more, depending on which path is followed.

There is significant variation in lung structure among individuals.* In fact, animal studies have demonstrated that biologic variability in respiratory tract anatomy is the dominant factor influencing the transit and deposition of airborne substances. A classic model of airway transition up to 23 generations, with associated features, is presented in Figure 1–2.

One characteristic of this branching, albeit sometimes irregular architecture, is that as air and its contents pass down the system, they travel first through a small number of high-volume tubes that connect to a larger number of smaller volume ducts. Consequences of this geometric progression are an increase in the surface area-to-volume ratio (because surface area decreases by an exponent of 2 while volume decreases by an

---

*The convention of referring to both lungs as "the lung" will generally be followed here.

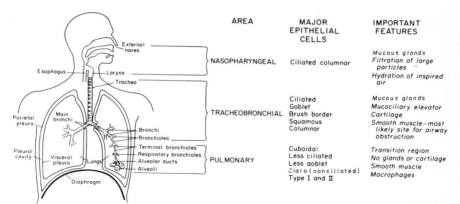

	AREA	MAJOR EPITHELIAL CELLS	IMPORTANT FEATURES
	NASOPHARYNGEAL	Ciliated columnar	Mucous glands Filtration of large particles Hydration of inspired air
	TRACHEOBRONCHIAL	Ciliated Goblet Brush border Squamous Columnar	Mucous glands Mucociliary elevator Cartilage Smooth muscle - most likely site for airway obstruction
	PULMONARY	Cuboidal Less ciliated Less goblet Clara (nonciliated) Type I and II	Transition region No glands or cartilage Smooth muscle Macrophages

Figure 1-1. Relationship of major components and features of the adult human respiratory system.

exponent of 3) and a decrease in flow rate due to redistribution of the air (Table 1–1).

The increase in surface area is significant for several reasons. First, one factor that influences the absorption of molecules across membranes in general is the surface area to which they are exposed. If all other parameters are the same, the deeper a substance can penetrate into the respiratory system, the more likely it will be taken up, because it will have access to a greater surface area. Second, the duration of exposure of a molecule to a membrane has a direct bearing on the quantity absorbed. Here, again, if deep penetration can be achieved, potential absorption may be enhanced due to decreased transit time and prolonged exposure.

The 2000-fold increase in cross-sectional area that occurs from bronchi to alveoli also has an important clinical correlate. It implies that obstructive airway disease must be quite disseminated in the terminal region (*e.g.*, as in diffuse fibrosis of the parenchyma) before it can be detected by measuring total airway resistance. Conversely, obstruction of higher regions (*e.g.*, as in bronchial asthma) will have a more significant effect on airway resistance. Detailed knowledge of the geometry of the respiratory apparatus is therefore central to a comprehensive understanding of

Table 1-1. Anatomic and Functional Characteristics of the Respiratory System*

Region (generation)	Number	Cross-Sectional Area	Flow Rate (cm/sec)
Main bronchi (1st)	2	3.2 cm²	180
Bronchioles (9th)	512	9.56 cm²	14
Respiratory bronchioles (17th)	1.3×10^5	300 cm²	0.9
Alveoli (23rd)	300×10^6	70 m²	0*

*These numbers are approximations, and vary according to source.

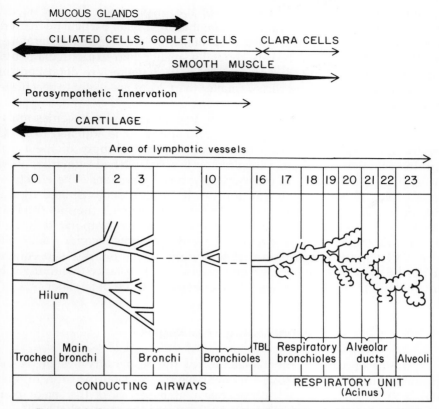

Figure 1–2. General architecture and associated characteristics of conducting and respiratory airways. (Modified from Weibel, E. R.: Morphometry of the Human Lung, Heidelberg, Springer-Verlag, 1963.)

particle or gas penetration, deposition, and clearance in the lung. However, only major features will be emphasized here.

Nasopharyngeal Region

The respiratory system is arbitrarily divided into several regions, or functional units. The first principal functional unit of the respiratory system that is conventionally designated is the nasopharyngeal. This region extends from the external nares to the trachea. It is lined with a mucous membrane composed primarily of ciliated columnar epithelial cells that are interspersed with mucus-secreting cells and glands. Mucus secreted by these glands and cells is carried by cilia to the back of the nasal cavity, where it can be swallowed or expectorated. Several hundred milliliters of mucus may be cleared and replaced each day in this manner.

The primary function of mucus within the nasopharyngeal region is to filter large airborne particles out of the inspired air. In this regard mucus is quite effective, removing more than 90% of all particulate matter. Virtually all particles over 10 μm in diameter are affected. Therefore, particles entering the trachea are generally smaller than 10 μm in diameter. Of these, most particles larger than 2 μm in diameter are deposited on the mucous layer; only particles smaller than 2 μm are likely to reach the terminal portion of the airway.

Within the nasopharyngeal region, incoming air also becomes moistened and warmed. The temperature of inspired air is adjusted to 37° C by the air-conditioning effect of the rich vascular supply of the nasal turbinates. Humidification of inspired air is accomplished primarily in the nasal passages through an outpouring of nasal secretions. The effectiveness of this humidification function can be readily demonstrated by the discomfort that occurs when a person breathes through the mouth. This process of moisturizing incoming air serves to lessen evaporative loss of water from the terminal respiratory bed and to hydrate incoming material. The latter function can have a significant effect on the subsequent deposition and transmembrane penetration of a substance (assuming it is hygroscopic). This process will be considered in more detail later.

Tracheobronchial Region

The second major functional unit of the respiratory system is the tracheobronchial. This region encompasses the trachea, the bronchi, and the bronchioles. The tracheobronchial region serves as the major conducting pathway between the nasopharynx and the terminal alveoli, and regulates the regional and generalized distribution of air in the lungs. In humans, the trachea is about 2 to 2.5 cm in diameter and about 11 cm long, and is composed of 16 to 20 U-shaped semirigid cartilaginous rings. On the posterior side, there is a thin trachealis muscle that extends between the open ends of the U and is shared by the esophagus. Contraction of this smooth muscle causes constriction of the trachea. Tracheal smooth muscle is often used as a model of airway smooth muscle, because it is mechanically similar to smooth muscle down to the sixth generation of bronchi.

Moving distally along the tracheobronchial region, the frequency of cartilaginous rings decreases. Bronchi, therefore, contain only a few terminal plates of cartilage, while bronchioles contain none. As cartilage decreases, there is an inversely proportional increase in smooth muscle. The presence of smooth muscle is the most important factor in determining the control of airway diameter. Respiratory smooth muscle tone is under autonomic control, principally parasympathetic (the significance of this relationship will be considered in more detail in succeeding chapters). Bronchi are nourished by the bronchial arteries that branch from the aorta, and are not part of the pulmonary circulation. Because they lack alveoli and are not exposed to pulmonary arterial blood, the bronchi cannot participate in gas exchange.

Next are the bronchioles, which lack cartilage, have limited smooth muscle, and are not held open by structural rigidity but by radial traction supplied by the elastic recoil of the surrounding parenchymal tissue. The tracheobronchial section is lined primarily with five types of epithelial cells and is coated with a thin 5-μm layer of mucus (Fig. 1–3). Ciliated epithelial cells are the predominant cells in this area. Some ciliated cells have become modified into secreting goblet cells (named for their shape). These cells contain the precursor of the mucin glycoprotein (mucigen), which is the principal component of mucus that is secreted. Goblet cells are not under nervous control but secretion can be stimulated by direct irritation. Ciliated cells normally outnumber goblet cells by about a 5:1 ratio.

As mentioned above, mucus secreted by goblet cells onto the surface of the airway functions to trap incoming particles and to protect the mucosa against dehydration. It also serves as the suspending vehicle for the movement of particles from the deep lung to the oral cavity. This is achieved via ciliary movement (mucociliary escalator) of the ciliated epithelial cells in the direction of the pharynx. In this way, undesirable particulate debris can be eliminated from the respiratory tract by expectoration from the oral cavity or by swallowing. It has been estimated that 10 to 100 ml of tracheobronchial mucus is produced each day, depending on circumstances.

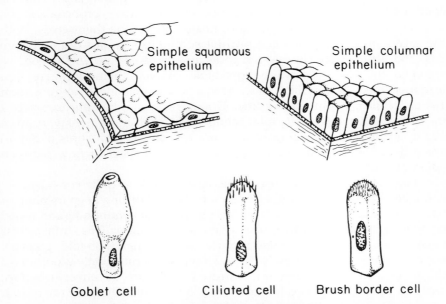

Figure 1–3. Examples of simple epithelia. (From Bowman, W. C., and Rand, M. J.: Textbook of Pharmacology, 2nd ed., Blackwell Scientific Publications, Oxford, 1980.)

Tracheobronchial submucosal glands, composed of clear mucous cells and stained serous cells, are also present in this area. Mucous glands represent about 12% of the wall thickness in mainstream bronchi, gradually diminishing to 0% in bronchioles. There are approximately 6000 in the human trachea, with the greatest concentration in the second to fifth generations of human bronchi (one gland/mm^2). Mucous glands have been estimated to have 100 times the volume of the goblet cells, and they probably secrete the most mucus in both healthy and disease states. They receive no sympathetic control but are innervated by parasympathetic nerves, which promote the secretion of their complex mucoproteins through duct systems that open like pores onto the airway surface.

Clara cells are found in terminal and respiratory bronchioles and appear to be secretory cells, which replace goblet cells in this area. Brush border cells, characterized by microvilli, are also present, and presumably specialize in absorption. Basal cells can also be observed, from which ciliated epithelial cells are believed to differentiate. The volume of air contained in the respiratory tract through the terminal bronchioles does not exchange gas with venous blood and is, therefore, effectively dead space in regard to gas exchange. This volume, the anatomic dead space, is normally about 150 ml in humans.

Pulmonary Region

The final unit of the respiratory system is the pulmonary, which is composed of the terminal bronchioles, the respiratory bronchioles, the alveolar ducts, the alveolar sacs and, finally, the alveoli themselves. With the exception of the terminal bronchioles, all these regions can exchange gas, and are collectively referred to as an acinus. About 200 alveoli are supplied by each respiratory bronchiole. Alveoli themselves are thin teacup-shaped, bellowslike sacs, with reported diameters ranging from 150 to 350 μm. Arranged in a line, 170 alveoli would be approximately 1 inch long. Estimates of the total number of alveoli in humans vary from 100 to 500 million. Interconnections between alveoli (the pores of Kohn) are believed to exist in the lung, and allow collateral air flow between adjacent portions.

The potential surface area of this terminal bed is quite considerable. Estimates from 35 m^2 during expiration to 140 m^2 during deep inspiration have been made. Approximately 75 m^2 is the most common figure, based on 300 million alveoli with a mean diameter of 250 μm. This surface is far larger than the skin in total area (averaging about 35-fold greater), approximating that of a tennis court. However, because only a portion of the alveolar surface is exposed to perfused capillaries, the effective surface area for gas exchange is estimated to be 35 to 40 m^2. The pulmonary unit serves primarily for the exchange of gases. However, by its very nature, the respiratory system also represents a significant portal for the introduction of either noxious or therapeutic agents. The lung can therefore be a primary site of organ toxicity, as well as a route of drug administration.

The alveoli themselves are lined with a single layer of flat epithelial cells about 0.1 to 0.5 μm thick, that form a thin barrier between the alveolar air and the interstitial capillary lumen. Each alveolus is surrounded by a dense plexus of approximately 1800 capillary segments (10 × 7 μm in area). This vascular arrangement represents the most dense capillary network in the body. If the 100 to 300 ml of blood in the pulmonary capillaries were to be spread over an alveolar surface of about 70 m², it would be equivalent to spreading 1 teaspoon of blood over a 1-m² surface. Thus, alveoli are intimately exposed to both the external and the internal environment and are, in a sense, in double jeopardy to substances therein.

MORPHOLOGY OF MAJOR LUNG CELLS

Morphologically, the lung may be divided into parenchymal (alveoli, alveolar ducts, and capillaries) and nonparenchymal tissue (conductive airways, conductive blood vessels, connective tissue structures, and pleura). These structures are composed of approximately 40 different cell types, as well as of connective tissue (collagen, elastin, and proteoglycans). Several reports have provided varying estimates of the relative contribution of parenchymal and nonparenchymal components to total lung mass. These estimates, which are based on animal studies, suggest that at least 86% of total lung cells are parenchymal in nature. These include alveolar type I (4 to 7.5%), alveolar type II (6 to 14.5%), endothelial (33 to 43%), and interstitial (32 to 43%) cells. The remaining cells are mainly ciliated, glandular, and blood vessel cells.

Additional data pertaining to the morphology of rat lung, which has been the most extensively studied, are shown in Table 1–2. Although the absolute values undoubtedly vary among species, as well as among

Table 1–2. Morphometric Characteristics of Rat Lung*

Cell Type	Compart-mental Volume Density	% Total Cells	Cell Volume (μm³)	Luminal Surface Area (μm²)
Type I	0.126	7.5	915	4518
Type II	0.097	14.5	366	62
Endothelial	0.264	43.0	336	946
Macrophages	0.039	3.2	665	
Interstitial	0.358	31.8	615	

*(From Haies, D. M., Gill, J., and Weibel, E. R.: Morphometric study of rat lung cells, 1. Numerical and dimensional characteristics of parenchymal cell population. Am. Rev. Resp. Dis., 123:535, 1980.)

animals, the relative relationships between categories will probably remain reasonably constant and provide a basis for extrapolation to human lung morphology.

Type I Alveolar Epithelial Cells

A schematic representation of the relationship of these parenchymal cells to other adjacent cells is shown in Figure 1–4. Lining each alveolus are two types of epithelial cells, which differ structurally and functionally. Type I alveolar epithelial cells are simple squamous (thin, flat) cells located at the bottom of the alveoli. Type I cells line more than 95% of the alveolar surface. They are relatively simple cells that contain very little cytoplasm and few organelles, and are less metabolically active than the neighboring type II cells. They do appear to have considerable smooth endoplasmic reticulum, however, which has been observed to proliferate under the stressful influence of toxic agents.

Because of their location and biochemical composition, type I cells are the parenchymal cells that are most susceptible to damage; this seems to be true whether toxins are inhaled or reach the lung via the bloodstream. Their main function is to provide a thin barrier to gaseous diffusion while consuming little oxygen themselves. The extent to which they represent a negligible barrier to diffusion is illustrated by the fact that the partial pressure of oxygen (Po_2) in pulmonary capillary blood (99 mm Hg) is almost identical with the Po_2 in alveolar air (100 mm Hg). However, alteration of the normal anatomic relationship of the type I cell to the capillary endothelial cell can have a significant effect. For example, thickening of either the alveolar or the capillary walls or separation of the membranes by edema fluid will effectively extend the necessary diffusion path and will attenuate the respiratory process.

Type II Alveolar Epithelial Cells

Located at the corners of the alveoli, and partly covered by cyto-plasmic extensions of type I cells, are epithelial type II cells. A relatively tight seal between these adjacent epithelial cells is presented by a contin-uous network of interconnecting filaments. In contradistinction to type I cells, type II cells have dense, well-defined cytoplasmic structures, includ-ing vacuoles, granular endoplasmic reticulum, Golgi apparatus, multives-icular bodies, and multilamellated inclusions. These cells are metabolically and mitotically active. Both type I and type II cells rest on a basement membrane composed of reticulin fibers.

Epithelial type II cells are believed to be the source of alveolar surfactant and are, therefore, secretory in nature. Surfactant is a surface tension-lowering material that regulates surface tension-related events at the air-liquid interface, which keeps the alveoli maximally distended for gas exchange (surfactant will be considered in more detail at the end of this chapter).

Within a given alveolus, type II cells tend to outnumber type I cells by approximately a 2:1 ratio. However, the total surface area of type I cells is approximately 35 times greater. Therefore, as mentioned above, type I cells comprise most of the alveolar epithelial barrier. Data from physiologic studies of the adult mammalian lung indicate that the alveolar epithelium forms the principal barrier to water-soluble solutes and behaves functionally as though it contains small water-filled pores, with a radius of 0.6 to 1.0 nm. This tight epithelial barrier is not absolute, however, because under certain circumstances transfer of protein to and from the alveolar lumen can occur.

Capillary Endothelial Cells

Immediately adjacent to the alveoli and separated by a basement membrane are pulmonary capillary endothelial cells. The lungs are believed to contain as many as 50% of all the endothelial cells in the body. Endothelial cells represent a continuous series of adjoining cytoplasmic compartments lining the vasculature. Adjacent endothelial cells are held in relatively close opposition along their lateral borders by intercellular junctions. However, there are a number of 4-nm wide intercellular clefts between adjacent membranes, so that the pulmonary endothelium tends to be "leakier" than the epithelium. In addition, the endothelium cell has a relatively high permeability to water, small ions, and uncharged metabolites, (e.g., urea and glucose). The endothelial cell body with its nucleus, mitochondria, endoplasmic reticulum, and Golgi apparatus is usually situated adjacent to the central connective tissue core of the alveolar wall.

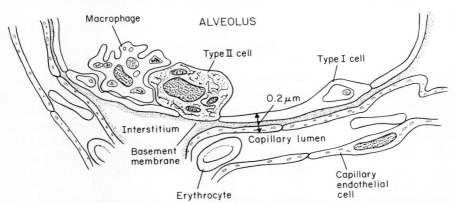

Figure 1–4. The basic structure of the alveolar-capillary unit. (From Bowman, W. C., and Rand, M. J.: Textbook of Pharmacology, 2nd ed., Blackwell Scientific Publications, Oxford, 1980.)

A striking feature of pulmonary capillary endothelial cells is the presence of a large number of vesicles, which are distributed among the plasma membrane (caveolae), cytoplasm, and basement membrane. However, membrane immediately adjacent to the alveolar epithelium is devoid of these vesicles to maintain a thin diffusion barrier. In fact, the diffusion distance from alveolar gas to red blood cells is smaller than a single red cell's diameter.

Results of studies in the rat indicate that endothelial cells have an individual cell surface area about 20% that of the epithelial type I cells. However, because there are about 5.7 times as many endothelial cells as type I cells, the endothelial surface would be about 16% greater than the alveolar surface. This would compute, in the human, to approximately 162 m^2, using an alveolar value of 140 m^2. However, this endothelial surface area value varies somewhat with that routinely found in the literature (120 m^2) for a 70-kg human.

Capillary endothelial cells are less active metabolically than type II cells but play an important role, as shall be seen, in the metabolism of certain amines, lipids, polypeptides, and nucleotides. As mentioned above, capillary endothelial cells represent less of a diffusion barrier than type I or II cells. In fact, the alveolar capillary endothelium has been shown to be a fairly porous structure, which allows the transport of various water-soluble molecules.

In general, the rates at which all substances penetrate endothelial cells, with the exception of the brain, are far greater than those at which these same materials cross epithelial tissue. The thickness of the capillary endothelial cell surface is approximately 0.1 µm. Because this is about the same thickness as the epithelial type I cell, the total gas exchange barrier of the alveolar-capillary unit is about 0.2 µm over the major part of the air-blood contact surface. Rates of absorption into or out of capillaries are usually determined by the oil:water coefficient for lipid-soluble substances and by the molecular size of lipid-insoluble substances.

Mesenchymal Cells

Within the interstitium and lying between the endothelial and epithelial cells are mesenchymal cells. These mesenchymal cells are primarily fibroblasts, which are surrounded by a connective tissue matrix. Fibroblast cells are primarily responsible for the synthesis of collagen, elastin fibers, and ground substance, which comprise this connective tissue matrix. Collagen is the major constituent of connective tissue in the lung, and constitutes 60 to 65% of the total extracellular mass. The remainder consists of elastic fibers (elastin and microfibrils, 35 to 40%) and proteoglycans (proteins and glycosaminoglycans [1 to 2%].

Collagen provides the principal architectural framework of the lung, and is a central component of the fibrous support scaffold. Fibroblast activity is, therefore, an important determinant of lung structure and function. There are certain situations, however, in which excessive fibroblast activity can lead to the deposition of abnormal amounts of collagen within the parenchyma (see Chap. 9). When this occurs, the diffusion and mechanical properties of the lung can change dramatically, producing hypoxia, dyspnea, and even death.

Macrophages

As indicated in Figure 1–4, there is another important type of cell within the alveoli in addition to the epithelial type I and II cells. These are the macrophages, which under scanning electron microscopy have a ruffled appearance, with few filopodia and a diameter of 12 to 20 μm. It has been calculated that there are between 3 and 15×10^6 macrophages/g of lung tissue in humans. This corresponds to a distribution of approximately 16 macrophages/alveolus. The turnover time of macrophages is about 24 hours, which results in the maintenance of a constant number of cells.

Macrophages are mobile and are metabolically very active, and possess phagocytic, microbicidal, and cytocidal activity. Macrophages are a major defense against inhaled toxicants and microorganisms, and represent the primary phagocytes of the lung. The origin of alveolar macrophages is unclear, although the most popular theory suggests that they are derived from precursor cells (promonocytes) in the bone marrow and from peripheral blood monocytes. Self-renewal via metabolic division has been postulated as an alternative explanation, but this hypothesis is less widely accepted.

Macrophages are concentrated within the alveolar region of the lung, in which they lie submerged beneath the layer of surfactant material in intimate contact with the membrane of epithelial cells. Most alveolar macrophages probably exit from the lungs by way of the mucociliary escalator (see Chap. 9).

Because of their phagocytic functions, alveolar macrophages necessarily have considerable enzymatic activity. They are rich in hydrolases and degradative enzymes, such as lysozyme, collagenase, and β-glucuronidase. They also have a relatively high concentration of the antioxidant enzyme superoxide dismutase as well as catalase. ATPase and AMPase have been identified on the surface of the cell facing the exterior (ectoenzymes).

Macrophages also contain many other enzymes. One of the most celebrated of these is α-antitrypsin (AAT); investigators feel that a deficit of AAT may be involved in the development of emphysema in the human. AAT can inhibit the activity of many proteolytic enzymes and, therefore, can protect tissues against their action. One proteolytic enzyme that has access to the lung is neutrophil elastase. If this enzyme is allowed to act unchecked, considerable structural and functional damage to the lung can occur via elastin breakdown. A certain small percentage of the human population (0.5%) has a profound deficiency of AAT resulting from a homozygous inheritance of two codominant autosomal genes. In such cases, activated unrestrained neutrophil elastase is believed to participate in the destruction of alveolar walls, leading to the development of the abnormally large air spaces that characterize emphysema.

Pulmonary macrophages also participate in the processing of inhaled antigenic materials, and thus may be active in pulmonary immunologic responses. In most cases, the material is rendered nonantigenic and is disposed of. A small portion of the antigen processed by macrophages is transferred to lymphocytes for immune sensitization. Sensitized T lymphocytes are believed to secrete lymphokines, which may participate in the "activation" of macrophages. Activated macrophages become enlarged and more aerobically active, increase their lysosomal enzyme content, and develop into more aggressive phagocytes.

Because macrophages represent one of the few barriers that exist to toxicants entering via the respiratory system, their normal function is important. Although not nearly enough information is known about their function in the lung, it is known that the phagocytic activity of these cells can be depressed by various factors including tobacco smoke, hypoxia, ethanol, and immunosuppressant drugs. These observations may help to explain the high frequency of respiratory infections noted in alcoholics and in those exposed to certain types of polluted air.

SURFACTANT

Alveoli may be considered to be a series of connected bubbles. Because the alveoli of the lung can vary in radius by a factor of 3 or 4, they are disproportionate in their volume. Under normal circumstances, the volume of the smaller alveoli would tend to empty into the larger because of the greater pressure in the former. If this occurred in the lung, there would be numerous collapsed small alveoli. Fortunately, a preventive mechanism exists. According to the formula of Laplace, the internal pressure of a bubble can be decreased either by reducing its surface tension or by increasing its radius. In the lung, the former alternative is achieved via a surface-active agent called surfactant. Surfactant is synthesized and secreted by type II alveolar epithelial cells. Secretion occurs by exocytosis and is probably continuous.

Chemistry and Function

Surfactant is not a specific chemical substance but is composed primarily of a mixture of at least seven phospholipids, of which approximately 80 to 85% is phosphatidylcholine. These phospholipids are prob-

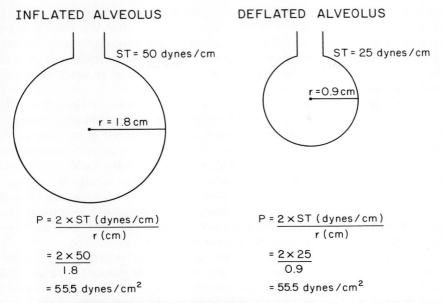

Figure 1–5. Relationship of radius(r) and surface tension (ST) to the internal pressure (P) of an alveolus. During deflation, surfactant lowers the surface tension to maintain constant internal pressure and to prevent collapse.

ably complexed to protein, which is added to the surfactant after its secretion into the alveoli. Alveolar surfactant has a short half-life (14 hours). Therefore, maintenance of adequate surfactant requires continuous synthesis.

Because there is normally a fixed quantity of surfactant for each alveolus, the surface tension-lowering effect is dependent on its quantitative relationship to alveolar surface area (Fig. 1–5). During inspiration, for example, the alveolus will expand and present an increased surface area, thereby decreasing the effect of surfactant. Conversely, during expiration, the alveolus has a tendency to collapse but, because the ratio of surfactant to surface area increases, the surface tension decreases, and the alveolus remains expanded.

These changes in surface tension stabilize the system and keep the various alveoli adequately inflated irrespective of their varying sizes. Alveoli can also remain dry and stable at low lung volumes, because surfactant lowers surface tension to values less than 10% of that of water or blood plasma. In the absence of surfactant, therefore, alveoli tend to fill with fluid or collapse.

Physiology

If surfactant is absent, alveoli will eventually collapse, leading to decreased lung compliance, decreased functional residual capacity, and decreased total lung capacity. Some situations in which surfactant is deficient will be discussed below. It is apparent that the alveoli must receive continuous vascular perfusion to maintain surfactant synthesis, which is why surfactant has been found to be absent from the lungs of deceased patients following open heart surgery when an artificial heart-lung machine was employed.

Surfactant normally appears in the lung of mammals at approximately the halfway point of gestation, and its synthesis then continues through-out the remainder of the term. Premature infants often have respiratory distress syndrome (RDS) caused by a deficit in surfactant. RDS also occurs with higher frequency in babies of diabetic mothers and in babies delivered by cesarean section. RDS was originally called hyaline membrane disease, a term that referred to the "glassy" look of the alveoli, which was caused by the presence of plasma that had leaked in. A proposed new treatment for RDS is the instillation of a lung surfactant preparation into the lung via the trachea. Clinical studies are currently being performed.

Several noteworthy observations suggest that pharmacologic inter-vention may, at some time in the future, be possible in high-risk RDS cases. For example, RDS is rarely observed in premature babies born to heroin addicts. The reason for this is unknown, but perhaps the most appealing explanation is that heroin may increase endogenous glucocor-ticoid secretion. In animal and human studies glucocorticoids have been found to enhance the production of surfactant, with attendant decreased mortality in premature neonates. There is also some evidence that indi-cates a lower incidence of RDS in premature babies from mothers who had taken oral contraceptives prior to pregnancy. These steroids may act by inducing the synthesis of enzymes involved in the production of surfactant. Studies in the rat also reveal that the thyroidal hormone L-thyroxine can stimulate the production of surfactant. This is believed to be the result of thyroid hormone binding to nuclear and cytoplasmic receptors in alveolar type II cells.

Surfactant synthesis or secretion (or both) is, in all probability, an important potential site for pneumotoxin or pharmacologic action. It has been suggested, for example, that alveolar silicolipoproteinosis, caused by inhalation of quartz crystals, may involve alteration of surfactant. In addition, *in vitro* studies have demonstrated an inhibition of surfactant synthesis by the pulmonary edemagenic agent 3-methylindole. Unfortu-nately, an inadequate number of studies have been carried out in this area, so there is little more than an intuitive feeling of concern.

It is known that drugs such as pilocarpine and β-adrenergic agonists, which have been reported to stimulate surfactant release, have been associated with interesting clinical and experimental observations. For example, a low incidence of RDS has been claimed in premature infants whose mothers had received a β-adrenergic agonist to prevent premature labor. Studies with isolated type II cells in culture indicate that β-adrenergic agonists can induce a slow 250 to 300% increase in surfactant secretion. The mechanism of action may involve stimulation of membrane-bound Na^+/K^+ ATPase, leading to alterations in ion distribution, membrane potential, and secretion. *In vivo* autoradiographic studies in the rat have demonstrated the presence of β-adrenergic binding sites in type II alveolar epithelial cells.

In addition to maintaining alveolar stability, surfactant may have other functions, including augmentation of the bactericidal capacity of alveolar macrophages and suppression of lymphocyte proliferation (immunosuppressant effect). The immunosuppressant effect is believed to be a consequence of the phospholipid component of surfactant. Here again, however, well-controlled systematic studies have not been carried out.

VASCULAR AND LYMPHATIC SYSTEMS

The lung is unique compared to other organ systems of the body in that it receives the entire cardiac output and is served with a dual blood vascular system. On the one hand there is the pulmonary circulation, which is a low-pressure, high-volume system that delivers nonoxygenated blood to the alveolar-capillary bed via the pulmonary arteries for gas exchange. In addition, the bronchial circulation has a relatively low volume of oxygenated blood at systemic pressure, which provides nutrients for the various pulmonary structures (lower trachea, bronchi, respiratory bronchioles). This blood originates from the aorta by way of the bronchial arteries. The result is that the lung has one of the highest relative blood flows per unit weight (Table 1–3).

Table 1–3. Relative Organ Perfusion Rates in Humans*

Organ	% Body Weight	Blood Flow (ml/min)	% Cardiac Output	Blood Flow (ml/min/100 g)
Well perfused				
Lung	1.2	5000	100	1000
Adrenals	0.02	25	1	550
Kidneys	0.4	1260	23	450
Thyroid	0.04	60	2	400
Liver				
Total	2	1350	25	75
(Via portal vein)		(1050)	(20)	(60)
Heart	0.4	252	5	70
Intestines	2	1050	20	60
Brain	2	750	15	55
Poorly perfused				
Skin	7	462	9	5
Skeletal muscle	40	840	16	3
Connective tissue	7			1
Fat	15	95	2	1

*(From Renwick, A. G.: Pharmacokinetics in toxicology. *In* Hayes, A. W. (ed.): Principles and Methods of Toxicology, New York, Raven Press, 1982, p. 663.)

Pulmonary Circulation

The pulmonary circulation starts in the pulmonary artery, emanating from the right ventricle, and ends in the left atrium. Movement of the blood in the pulmonary circulation occurs through a transition of arteries with declining diameter and increasingly muscular walls. However, pulmonary arteries have much thinner walls and muscular coats, in proportion to diameter, than do systemic arteries. They are, therefore, more expandable than the systemic vascular bed. The pulmonary vasculature, because of this distensibility, can accommodate variations in circulatory load with little change in pressure. This reduced muscularity can, nevertheless, achieve vasoconstriction because of the lower intravascular pressure. Eventually, the blood traverses the arterial tree to reach arterioles of approximately 70 μm in diameter, from which the blood enters the capillary bed.

In humans, lung capillaries have a diameter of approximately 6 to 15 μm, with a total length of approximately 1500·miles. They hold approximately 215 ml of blood. Pulmonary capillaries serve as the site for the two-way transfer of gases, nutrients, toxins, hormones, and drugs. Not all the capillary bed carries active blood flow at all times. During periods of exercise-induced increased cardiac output, for example, these nonfunctioning capillaries are recruited. Postcapillary oxygenated blood flows through venules with diameters less than 100 μm, eventually reaching pulmonary veins in the interlobular septa. Venous outflow continues via the superior and inferior pulmonary veins of each lung, which connect directly with the left atrium.

Pulmonary capillary hydrostatic pressure is relatively low, in the range of 6 to 10 mm Hg. Because this is lower than the colloidal osmotic pressure of plasma (25 to 30 mm Hg), any water present in the alveoli or interstitium becomes quickly absorbed into the blood (Starling's principle of transcapillary fluid movement). This is a very effective mechanism for keeping air spaces dry and for preventing interstitial edema. If pulmonary pressure rises above plasma colloidal osmotic pressure, fluid movement will be in the direction of the alveoli and the interstitium. Such a condition will produce pulmonary edema, and can result in a significant reduction in the exchange of oxygen and carbon dioxide. An elevation in pulmonary capillary pressure is common in congestive heart failure and myocardial infarction, in which blood backs up in the capillary network.

Lymph Drainage

As mentioned previously, pulmonary capillary endothelial cells have a certain degree of porosity, which results in a continuous flow of fluid from the vascular system toward the interstitium of the lung. If this process were allowed to progress indefinitely, fluid and protein would accumulate in the interstitium, leading to edema and to altered hemody-namics and gas exchange. Fortunately, under normal circumstances, the interstitium is efficiently drained of this vascular transudate via the lymphatic capillary system. The significance of this process can be illus-trated by data obtained from studies of sheep. In this species, lymphatic flow amounts to 5 to 8 ml/hour. The absence of this mechanism would effectively double the air-blood barrier in approximately 1 hour. It is estimated that lung lymphatic flow is approximately 20 ml/hour in a normal 70-kg human.

Within the pulmonary lymphatic system, fluid, proteins, and cells (e.g., macrophages) are taken up and moved through a series of collecting vessels interspersed with nodes. Unidirectional lymph flow is maintained by a system of conical valves. These lymph nodes function to filter out antigens and other foreign substances from the lymph before it is returned to the systemic circulation via the thoracic and other ducts. Damage to the pulmonary lymphatic system by inflammation, neoplasia, or fibrosis can obviously result in interstitial edema and in increased airway resis-tance.

INNERVATION

The lung receives innervation from both the parasympathetic and the sympathetic divisions of the autonomic nervous system. Parasympathetic outflow provides the excitatory innervation to pulmonary airways (smooth muscle) and glands. This efferent nerve supply is by way of the vagus nerves, and uses acetylcholine as the neurotransmitter (cholinergic). The status of normal pulmonary smooth muscle tone indicates parasympa-thetic dominance. The vagus nerves are, therefore, responsible for the maintenance of airway tone.

Direct stimulation of the parasympathetic fibers or the administration of cholinergic agents will produce diffuse airway constriction and glan-dular secretion. The location of airway constriction corresponds to the distribution of cholinergic fibers. Tracheal and bronchial smooth muscle are most affected, whereas alveolar ducts and terminal bronchioles are unaffected.

In comparison to the parasympathetic pathway, the sympathetic nerve supply to the airways is not as well characterized but appears to be of minor importance. It is known that postganglionic fibers emanating from the stellate ganglia enter the lung and, in close association with postganglionic parasympathetic fibers, ramify throughout the smooth muscle from trachea to respiratory bronchioles. The presence of sympa-thetic fibers in lower regions is the result of innervation of blood vessels. The density of sympathetic innervation to the airways is species-depend-ent, being high in the cat and the calf, lower in the guinea pig, and insignificant in the rabbit and the rat. Activation of the sympathetic innervation to lung smooth muscle results in airway dilation through the release of norepinephrine.

There is some disagreement, however, as to whether or not this is a direct effect. A postulated model suggests that sympathetic fibers actually function as presynaptic inhibitors of the parasympathetic fibers (via α_2 receptors). Release of acetylcholine is thereby reduced, and bronchial tension is relaxed. Two classes of adrenergic receptors have been identified on cell surfaces, the α- and β-adrenergic receptors, with the α class being further subdivided into α_1 and α_2 types of receptors. The α_1-adrenergic receptors are involved in mobilization of calcium across cell membranes, and are blocked by compounds such as verapamil. The α_2-adrenergic receptors are coupled to adenylate cyclase and have inhibitory action. Known α_2 agonists are clonidine and *p*-aminoclonidine; α_2 antagonists include yohimbine and tolazoline. The β-adrenergic receptors are coupled to adenylate cyclase activity and have stimulatory action (see below).

Smooth Muscle Contraction

The mechanism for smooth muscle contraction appears to involve an interaction between acetylcholine and muscarinic receptors on the surface of the smooth muscle cells to activate guanylate cyclase (Fig. 1–6). The

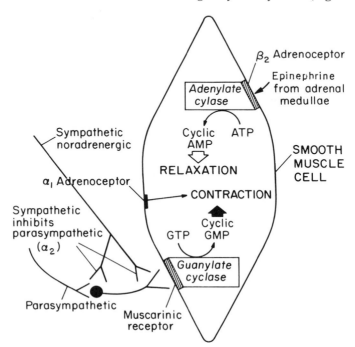

Figure 1–6. Hypothetic relationship between adrenergic and cholinergic "second messengers" in controlling the contractile activity of airway smooth muscle cells. (From Bowman, W. C., and Rand, M. J.: Textbook of Pharmacology, 2nd ed., Blackwell Scientific Publications, Oxford, 1980.)

result is an increase in the intracellular concentration of the "second messenger," cyclic GMP, which in some way provides more calcium ions for the contractile process. Because the nucleotide and the ion frequently function as interrelated second messengers, they have been termed "synarchic messengers." The tone of the smooth muscle becomes increased as myosin light chain kinase is activated, leading to phosphorylation of myosin and interaction with actin. Inhibition of parasympathetic activity or activation of adrenergic receptors, as shall be seen, can produce smooth muscle relaxation in the airway.

Smooth Muscle Relaxation

Most adrenergic receptors present in airway smooth muscle are of the β_2 classification. The ratio of β_2 receptors to β_1 receptors has been determined to be approximately 3:1. These β_2 receptors mediate bronchodilation and are responsive to epinephrine and other β_2 agonists. However, they do not receive direct sympathetic innervation. Studies in the dog indicate that β-adrenergic receptor density and responsiveness are substantially higher near the cervical end of the trachea than near the thoracic end. Autoradiographic studies in the rat indicate that β receptors are diffusely distributed within the lung, and are present in bronchi, bronchioles, alveoli, capillaries, and large blood vessels.

The mechanism that produces bronchodilation appears to involve the activation of membrane-bound adenylate cyclase by circulating agonists. The resultant elevation in intracellular cyclic AMP concentration is believed to decrease the availability of free calcium ions for the contractile process, thereby reducing smooth muscle tone. The mechanism may involve binding of calcium to the sarcoplasmic reticulum, uptake and sequestration of calcium by mitochondria, or actual efflux of calcium from the cell. A low level of intracellular calcium antagonizes actin-myosin interaction.

Direct sympathetic innervation through which norepinephrine produces relaxation by acting on β_2-receptors is also possible, and may explain the effect of some drugs. The presence of α receptors subserving bronchoconstriction can be demonstrated with exogenous norepinephrine after the β_2 receptors have been blocked with an appropriate antagonist.

Afferent Nerves

Afferent sensory fibers originate in the epithelium of airways, muscle, submucosa, and interalveolar spaces, and terminate in the vagal nuclei. There are three main types of afferents in the lung and airways: irritant fibers, which play an important role in various reflexes (*e.g.*, cough, bronchoconstriction); stretch receptors, which are involved with normal respiration; and J receptors (juxtapulmonary capillary receptors), which are believed to lie in the alveolar walls where they are adjacent to pulmonary capillaries. These J receptors can be stimulated by factors that increase pulmonary interstitial pressure, such as pulmonary congestion, edema, microembolism, pneumonia, and chemical factors such as inhalation of irritants. J receptors are, therefore, accessible through both the pulmonary circulation and the airway. Activation of J receptors produces rapid shallow breathing, with reduced tidal volume.

SELECTED REFERENCES

Burrows, B., et al. (ed.): Normal physiology. In Respiratory Disorders—A Pathophysiologic Approach, 2nd ed. Chicago, Year Book Medical Publishers, 1983, pp. 3–65.

Butler, C.: Respiratory anatomy and histology. In Gong, H., and Drage, C. W. (eds.): The Respiratory System: A Core Curriculum, Norwalk, Appleton-Century-Crofts, 1980, pp. 3–12.

Freedman, B. J.: The functional geometry of the bronchi. Bull. Physiopathol. Resp. 8:545, 1972.

Gill, J.: Comparative morphology and structure of the airways. In Witschi, H., and Nettesheim, P. (eds.): Mechanisms in Respiratory Toxicology, Vol. 1, Boca Raton, CRC Press, 1982, pp. 3–25.

Haies, D., Gill, J., and Weibel, E. R.: Morphometric study of rat lung cells. I. Numerical and diversional characteristics of parenchymal cell population. Am. Rev. Resp. Dis. 123:533, 1981.

Jeffery, P. K.: The normal structure of bronchial epithelium. In Bonsignore, G., and Cumming, G. (eds.): The Lung in its Environment, Vol. 6, Life Sciences, New York, Plenum Press, 1982, pp. 57–72.

Richardson, J.: Nerve supply to the lungs. Am. Rev. Resp. Dis. 119:785, 1979.

Weibel, E. R.: How does lung structure affect gas exchange? Chest 83:657, 1983.

CHAPTER 2

Factors Affecting Respiration

THE RESPIRATORY PROCESS

General Considerations

The primary respiratory function of the lung is the provision of an interface between the environmental atmosphere and the internal vascular system to supply oxygen (O_2) for metabolism and to permit the exit of carbon dioxide (CO_2), a product of that metabolism. However, humans exist in a gaseous atmosphere, whereas their component metabolizing cells function in a fluid milieu. Thus, O_2 and CO_2 must be transferred between the gas and liquid phases.

The process of respiration involves an interplay of various sensory and motor factors, and each of these factors represents a possible site for toxin or drug action. The respiratory process serves to regulate not only arterial blood concentrations of O_2 and CO_2 but hydrogen ion (H^+) as well, within prescribed limits. The lung performs this role in three major ways: by having a large surface area for gas exchange; by presenting a thin barrier to diffusion; and by having a high blood flow.

For efficient gas exchange and oxygenation of blood to occur, blood perfusion volume and alveolar ventilation should ideally be matched. Under normal circumstances the volume of gas exchange is approximately 4 liters/minute, which is similar to the approximate blood volume perfusing the alveoli (5 liters/minute). The overall ventilation:perfusion ratio for the lung is, therefore, in the range of 0.8 to 1.0. Studies in humans using radioactive xenon indicate, however, that both ventilation and blood flow are nonuniform in the lungs of normal patients. The highest blood flow rates are seen near the bottom and decrease with distance up the lung. The converse is true of ventilation. Therefore, there exists a great variability in the ventilation-perfusion relationship in different areas of the lung.

Oxygen Uptake

The driving force behind the movement of a gas is its partial pressure (measured in torr, or mm Hg). Partial pressure is dependent on the concentration of a gas and its kinetic energy. Mathematically, partial pressure is a set fraction of the total pressure when several gases exist in the same volume. For example, the partial pressure of O_2 (PO_2) in dry inspired air at sea level is $0.21 \times 760 = 160$ mm Hg. At an altitude of 5000 feet, the fractional composition of O_2 would remain 0.21, but, because the total atmospheric pressure would be reduced to 632 mm Hg, the ambient PO_2 would be 132.5 mm Hg. Water vapor can also exert pressure. For example, in alveolar air, the fractional concentration of O_2 is reduced to 0.14 by water vapor, so its partial pressure is reduced to approximately 100 mm Hg.

The rate of diffusion of O_2 and CO_2 across the alveolar and pulmonary capillary membranes and across the capillary membranes in tissue is proportional to their partial pressure gradients. Therefore, oxygen moves from alveolar air to blood because the PO_2 is higher in alveolar air (100 mm Hg) than in venous blood (43 mm Hg). Conversely, CO_2 passes from venous blood (47 mm Hg) to alveolar air (essentially 0 mm Hg) for the same reason.

The passage of an erythrocyte through a pulmonary capillary has a duration of about 0.75 second. During the first 0.25 second, O_2 equilibration is reached. Therefore, there is a threefold factor of safety for oxygen diffusion, and capillary transit time could be shortened by 67% before dysequilibrium would be expected. The partial pressure of CO_2 (PCO_2) for erythrocyte and plasma falls more slowly, with equilibrium being reached after 0.6 to 0.7 and 0.4 second, respectively. This indicates that the safety factor for CO_2 diffusion is less than that for O_2.

OXYGEN TRANSPORT

Binding to Hemoglobin

The O_2 content of blood is determined not only by its relative O_2 tension, however. Other factors such as hemoglobin content, temperature, CO_2 content, and pH are also influential. The absence of hemoglobin, for example, is incompatible with life; because at an alveolar PO_2 of 100 mm Hg only 0.3 ml of O_2 will be dissolved in 100 ml of blood as a simple solution. This amount of O_2 is inadequate for the maintenance of complex life forms. However, during the process of evolution, O_2-binding pigments were incorporated into our hematopoietic system to compensate for this shortcoming.

In vertebrates, the respiratory pigment is iron-containing hemoglobin. Each 100 ml of blood contains approximately 15 g of hemoglobin, which carries 1.34 ml O_2/g of hemoglobin. The presence of hemoglobin, therefore, increases the oxygen-carrying capacity of blood to approximately 20.4 ml O_2/ ml blood (20.1 + 0.3). However, at the normal P_{O_2} of the alveoli (100 mm Hg) hemoglobin is 97% saturated, and each 100 ml of pulmonary venous blood contains approximately 19.5 ml of O_2 in combination with hemoglobin and 0.3 ml in simple solution.

The relationship of P_{O_2} to hemoglobin saturation with O_2 is an interesting one. The hemoglobin molecule is basically a receptor for oxygen. It is a tetramer composed of four units of an iron-containing porphyrin (heme) and an associated polypeptide (globin). Each atom of iron can combine with one molecule of O_2 (oxygenation). Sequential binding of the iron atoms with O_2 produces a successive increase in the affinity of the remaining iron atoms for O_2 (cooperative binding). This increased affinity is produced by conformational changes in the remaining protein subunits of the molecule. Increasing the P_{O_2} will, therefore, tend to increase not only the degree but the rate at which hemoglobin becomes saturated.

If a plot is made of the degree of blood saturated with O_2 as a function of P_{O_2}, a characteristic curve is obtained. This is usually referred to as the O_2 dissociation curve, although the term "association curve" would, in fact, be more appropriate in regard to binding. As seen in Figure 2–1, the binding of O_2 to hemoglobin has the usual sigmoidal shape of a drug receptor binding relationship. In fact, the terms "concentration" and "binding" can be substituted for P_{O_2} and percent saturation, respectively.

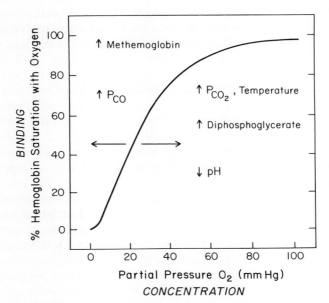

Figure 2–1. Oxygen dissociation curve of human blood.

The term "dissociation" has been traditionally used because principles related to the release of oxygen from hemoglobin have been physiologically more important, historically. An important physiologic correlate of the O_2 association-dissociation curve is that arterial P_{O_2} can fall significantly before the O_2 content or saturation of the blood shows an appreciable decrease. For example, if arterial P_{O_2} is decreased by 45%, oxygen saturation is decreased by only 10.5%. This relationship, therefore, tends to maintain an adequate oxygen supply.

Alterations in Hemoglobin Binding

As mentioned above, factors such as temperature, CO_2 content, and pH can alter the O_2 content of blood. Under normal circumstances CO_2 and pH are the most important, and are intimately related. Their roles and relationship will be briefly discussed.

CO_2 is transported in the blood in three forms: 5% is in solution in blood plasma; 5% is carried as carbamino groups of hemoglobin; and 90% exists as bicarbonate ion. The bicarbonate ion is formed primarily as a result of the influence of carbonic anhydrase in red cells:

$$CO_2 + H_2O \xrightleftharpoons{\text{Carbonic anhydrase}} H_2CO_3 \rightleftharpoons HCO_3^- + H^+$$

The carbonic acid thus formed then dissociates, and the bicarbonate diffuses out of the erythrocyte to re-establish equilibrium conditions. Excess CO_2 will, therefore, tend to increase H^+ concentration (decrease in pH). The hydrogen ions then interact with hemoglobin, leading to an alteration in charge distribution, conformational change, and a decrease in its affinity for O_2.

As with any drug-receptor interaction, decreased affinity is manifested in a shift to the right of the binding curve (Fig. 2–1). In the case of CO_2, the shift to the right of the curve is referred to as the Bohr effect. This effect plays an important fundamental role in normal physiology by facilitating O_2 delivery to tissues, because the higher CO_2 concentration in tissue will decrease the affinity of hemoglobin for O_2 and promote its dissociation and diffusion.

Another physiologic mechanism used to maximize oxygen delivery to tissues is the production of the metabolite 2,3-diphosphoglycerate (DPG). During periods of hypoxia, anaerobic glycolysis increases in erythrocytes, leading to an increase in DPG. The excess DPG then binds to the β-chain subunits of deoxygenated hemoglobin, reducing their ability to combine with oxygen and thereby facilitating oxygen availability. This alteration in affinity is reflected in a shift of the dissociation curve to the right.

If blood is stored for a significant period of time, DPG concentrations decrease. This results in an increased affinity for O_2 binding to hemoglobin, as reflected in a shift to the left of the dissociation curve. Less oxygen will therefore be available for diffusion. This may be an important consideration prior to transfusion of blood, because "old" blood will have less of a tendency to release oxygen. On the other hand, part of the tissue reparative properties of glucocorticoids may involve increased availability of oxygen to injured tissue. It has been reported, for example, that prednisone can significantly increase the red cell content of DPG.

Under normal circumstances, up to 2% of hemoglobin may be in its methemoglobin form (Fe^{3+}; oxidized). Methemoglobin levels can increase as the result of hemoglobinopathies, defects in erythrocyte metabolism, and the toxic effect of drugs or chemicals (most cases). If high enough levels of methemoglobin (30 to 40%) are found, symptoms of anoxia can result. The anoxia results both from a decrease in the oxygen-carrying capacity of hemoglobin and from an increased affinity of the remaining heme groups for oxygen. The result is a shift to the left of the oxygen association-dissociation curve, with impaired delivery of oxygen to tissues.

Methemoglobinemia can be produced by many aromatic substances containing amino or nitro groups (Table 2–1). Most of these substances undergo metabolic transformations in the liver, yielding products with the ability to oxidize hemoglobin. The most common cause of methemoglobinemia is accidental or deliberate overdosage with aniline-containing analgesic drugs. Industrial poisoning may occur from inhalation of the vapors or from absorption of these chemicals through the skin.

In cases in which dangerous levels of methemoglobin have been formed, the goal of therapy is to accelerate the rate of Fe^{3+} reduction to Fe^{2+}. Because the normal rate of reversion is only about 12%/hour, the administration of reducing agents such as ascorbic acid or methylene blue will accelerate conversion more rapidly.

In addition to the "normal" constituents of the atmosphere, the lung can also be exposed to any toxicants that are present as gases. Therefore, the same factors that promote an efficient exchange of oxygen and carbon dioxide can also facilitate the absorption of respirable gaseous toxicants (e.g., respiratory rate, effective surface area, blood flow, and partial pressure). Gases such as N_2, N_2O, H_2, and He are simple asphyxiants that, if their partial pressures are high enough, can decrease available oxygen in the air. Serious adverse effects can be produced when the available oxygen concentration is lowered to less than 10% (21% is normal).

Carbon monoxide (CO) is the classic chemical asphyxiant. It has an affinity for hemoglobin oxygen-binding sites 100 to 200 times greater than oxygen. The net result is a significant reduction in oxygen-carrying capacity. Furthermore, the formation of carboxyhemoglobin shifts the dissociation curve of the remaining normal hemoglobin to the left, so that the release of bound oxygen to the tissues is decreased. CO poisoning, therefore, has the dual effects of successfully competing with free O_2 for

Table 2–1. Some Amino and Nitro Compunds that Produce Methemoglobinemia

Aromatic Compounds	Aliphatic and Inorganic Compounds
Aniline	Sodium nitrite
Anilinoethanol	Hydroxylamine
Phenacetin	Dimethylamine
Acetanilid	Nitroglycerine
Methylacetanilid	Amyl nitrite
Hydroxylacetanilid	Ethyl nitrite
Sulfanilamide	Bismuth subnitrate
Sulfathiazole	Ammonium nitrate
Sulfisomidine	Potassium nitrate
Phenylenediamine	
Aminophenol	
Toluenediamine	
α-Naphthylamine	
p-Aminopropriophenone	
Phenylhydroxylamine	
Toluhydroxylamine	
Nitrobenzene	
Dinitrobenzene	
Trinitrotoluene	
Nitrosobenzene	
p-Nitroaniline	
Tetraline	
Pyridine	
Benzoquinone	
Hydroquinone	
Thionine	
Benzocaine	
Phenylhydrazine	

binding sites and of retarding the release of bound O_2. The treatment of CO poisoning is artificial ventilation with oxygen that competes with CO for hemoglobin-binding sites. Death can occur following a 1-hour exposure to 0.35% carbon monoxide.

TOXIC GASES

Absorption

Unlike the exchanges of O_2 and CO_2 in the alveoli, the absorption of certain toxic gases can occur throughout the entire respiratory system. The principal factors determining the absorption of a toxic gas are its concentration, water solubility, and hygroscopic nature (the latter two features will be dealt with below). Pathologic response by the pulmonary system can be acute or chronic, or the lung can simply act as a conduit and the injury can occur elsewhere in the body.

Distribution

Before a toxic gas can produce cell damage, it must at least go farther than either the upper airway mucus or the alveolar surfactant layer. Some toxic gas can dissolve in the mucous layer to be detoxified by mucociliary removal. If the concentration and duration of exposure to an inhaled toxic gas are sufficient to shift the toxicant across mucous and surfactant layers by mass action, toxicity to adjacent lung cells can occur. Any of the cells between the site of absorption and the site of entrance into the vascular system can be affected.

Toxic gases that penetrate the mucous lining of the upper airway will primarily contact the goblet, ciliated, and brush border epithelial cells. Ciliated cells appear to be the most sensitive of the three types, which is not surprising because they have more primitive intracellular machinery. The degree of injury to ciliated cells can range from the loss of a few cilia to death of the cell. As a result, ciliated cell debris can often be identified in expectorated mucus.

If a toxic gas reaches the alveolus, its uptake is treated basically like that of O_2. While in this region, type I cells will be especially prone to injury. Alveolar macrophages can also be injured and die. Release of their intracellular enzymes can destroy the alveolar septa and contribute to the development of emphysema.

RESPIRATORY STIMULANT DRUGS

In most circumstances in which artificial ventilation is required, mechanical ventilation has been found to be the safest and most effective means. Infrequently, however, it may be deemed undesirable to ventilate a patient mechanically because of fears related to weaning from the respirator and the risks of intubation. In such situations, respiratory stimulant drugs may provide a possible alternative for maintaining gas exchange until the acute respiratory failure has subsided. There are a number of potential sites for drug action within the respiratory process. Ventilation, for example, is composed of afferent, efferent, and central components, all of which can be affected in one manner or another (Fig. 2–2).

It would be extremely helpful if drugs existed that could selectively stimulate the breathing process in humans. Unfortunately, no such drugs are known. There are a group of drugs optimistically referred to as analeptics (restorative), which are occasionally used for such a purpose. It should be understood, though, that these pharmacologic agents are basically only nonspecific central nervous system (CNS) stimulants with secondary respiratory activation. Analeptics may act directly on the medulla to stimulate breathing or may act indirectly to stimulate carotid chemoreceptors. Their central stimulation is dose-dependent, and may

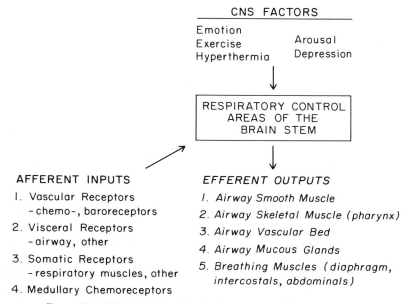

Figure 2–2. Afferent, CNS, and efferent components in ventilation.

culminate in convulsions. In fact, some are often used to produce convulsions in animal experiments to screen for anticonvulsant drugs.

The stimulation of respiration produced by these analeptics is transient, lasting for only about 5 to 10 minutes. If such a brief response can be of value, then the use of an appropriate drug may be warranted. However, very few clinical situations have been identified in which this is the case. One such instance may be the injudicious use of oxygen, in which the acute use of analeptics may effect some counteractive benefit. There is no compelling evidence indicating that chronic administration of analeptics affords any real therapeutic advantages in any situation. In fact, repeated doses may intensify CNS depression.

Doxapram

Currently, the safest and most accepted analeptic is doxapram (Fig. 2–3). Doxapram appears to stimulate both the medullary respiratory center and carotid bodies. Animal studies indicate, however, that most of the respiratory stimulant effect is accounted for by its action on the carotid bodies, and that large doses are required for a central effect. Its role in respiratory therapeutics is controversial, and further evaluation of its potential in hypoventilation syndromes is needed. The limited studies that have been done purport to demonstrate that doxapram may have the

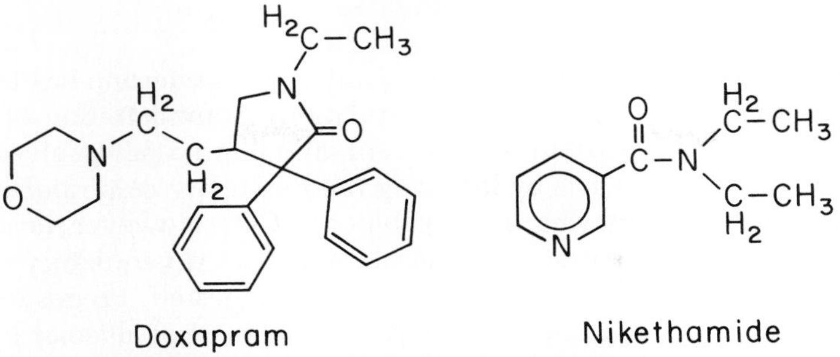

Doxapram   Nikethamide

Figure 2–3. Structures of two respiratory stimulants.

following effects: prevent or reverse narcotic and anesthetic-induced ventilatory depression; hasten arousal during postoperative recovery; and help to initiate respiration in neonates.

However, the definitive clinical usefulness of doxapram in these situations has not been established. In addition, doxapram should not be used to stimulate ventilation in patients severely intoxicated with general depressants, because controlled ventilation and standard supportive therapy have been shown to be superior. There may be some short-term benefit achieved with doxapram in alleviating respiratory depression induced by oxygen therapy in carefully selected cases.

Doxapram is available as a 2% solution, and is administered either as a bolus or by continuous infusion. It has sometimes been used continuously over a period of hours or days in the hope of providing sustained ventilatory stimulation. Reported side effects include coughing, nausea, vomiting, restlessness, hypertension, tachycardia, cardiac arrhythmias, muscle rigidity, and convulsions. Doxapram is contraindicated in patients with convulsive disorders, hypertension, cerebral edema, hyperthyroidism, pheochromocytoma, and those taking monoamine oxidase inhibitors or adrenergic agents.

Nikethamide

The only other analeptic worthy of note here is nikethamide (Fig. 2–3). Like doxapram, it acts by stimulating the medullary centers and the carotid bodies. It is a potent general and respiratory stimulant. Its only remaining use is occasionally as a respiratory stimulant in chronic bronchitis. When used, it is given intravenously by intermittent injections. Side effects can include sweating, nausea, vomiting, coughing, flushing of the skin and, if the dose is high enough, epileptic seizures followed by CNS depression. Nikethamide has only a minor role, and doxapram is preferable because of its wider margin of safety.

Hormones

Of the various steroid hormones studied, progesterone has produced the most interest for its effects on ventilation. Administration of progesterone causes an increase in minute ventilation and a fall in alveolar CO_2 tension. The hormone acts by lowering the medullary respiratory center's threshold and by increasing its excitability to CO_2. However, an action at peripheral chemoreceptors, resulting in an increased ventilatory response to hypoxia rather than to CO_2, has also been suggested. Progesterone has been reported to have clinical utility in the treatment of alveolar hypoventilation, in the respiratory depression of metabolic alkalosis, in improvement of ventilation in pulmonary emphysema, and in the pickwickian syndrome.

Other hormones, including adrenocorticotropic hormone (ACTH), thyroxine, and catecholamines, have also been reported to affect respiration. ACTH and thyroxine are believed to increase the excitability of the respiratory center, whereas catecholamines may cause a reflex increase in ventilation by decreasing perfusion of the carotid bodies. Ventilation in humans can be increased by isoproterenol and albuterol. The effect is believed to be β receptor-mediated in the carotid body, resulting in increased responsiveness to hypoxia and hypercapnia. Fortunately, β blockers such as propranolol cause minimal reductions in ventilatory drive in humans. There is little danger, therefore, that patients will be harmed because of the respiratory side effects of β-adrenergic antagonist drugs, as opposed to their effects on the airways (see Chap. 4).

RESPIRATION SUPPRESSION

In certain circumstances it is desirable to suppress unwanted, irregular spontaneous ventilation so that effective, regular artificial ventilation can be achieved. When appropriate, this may be achieved by the use of oxygen, morphine, or neuromuscular blocking agents.

Oxygen and Morphine

Exposure to 100% oxygen for not more than 10 minutes can inactivate the hypoxic chemoreceptor drive so that the patient's own breathing is eliminated, and the patient may be artificially ventilated.

Morphine sulfate suppresses respiration by depressing the activity of the medullary respiratory center. Under normal circumstances, this is an undesirable feature that contraindicates its use in patients with compromised breathing. Effective suppression of ventilation can occur within 10 minutes of administration of a 5-mg intravenous dose, although a series of 5-mg doses every 10 minutes up to a total dosage of 20 mg may be necessary in a minority of cases. Potential side effects include nausea and vomiting, hypotension, and gaseous distention of the bowel (caused by decreased peristalsis). Addiction liability is not a concern because of the brief duration of therapy.

Neuromuscular Blocking Drugs

Neuromuscular blocking drugs can block the transmission of motor nerve impulses to skeletal muscles by competitive blockade of acetylcholine receptors (*e.g.*, *d*-tubocurarine) or by persistent depolarization (*e.g.*, succinylcholine). They are often used as an adjunct in surgical anesthesia to produce muscular relaxation, making manipulation of muscular tissues much easier with a lower depth of anesthesia, and postanesthesia recovery time is therefore reduced. In respiratory therapy there are two primary applications for neuromuscular blocking drugs: endotracheal intubation and the prevention of spontaneous breathing in a patient on a mechanical ventilator.

The use of these drugs should only be carried out under close supervision because, in addition to their effect on respiration, each has significant side effects. Conscious patients should definitely be tranquilized or sedated before receiving these blocking drugs (because the experience is very unpleasant), and should not be left unattended.

When an appropriate dose of *d*-tubocurarine is injected intravenously (the route of choice), the onset of effects is evident in 3 to 5 minutes. Small rapidly moving muscles are affected first, followed by limb, neck, trunk, intercostal and, finally, diaphragm muscles. The duration of action of *d*-tubocurarine is approximately 30 to 60 minutes. Recovery of muscles usually occurs in the reverse order to that of their paralysis, so that the diaphragm is ordinarily the first to regain function.

In case of overdose, artificial respiration may be sufficient, although the cholinesterase inhibitor neostigmine methylsulfate (given intravenously) should be available as an antidote, as well as atropine sulfate to antagonize excess muscarinic effects produced by the neostigmine. General anesthetics such as ether, cyclopropane, halothane, and methoxyflurane can potentiate the effect of *d*-tubocurarine. Ether can, in fact, reduce the dosage of *d*-tubocurarine used for endotracheal intubation to 10%.

The major danger associated with *d*-tubocurarine use is the rapid injection of large doses. Under these circumstances, histamine can be liberated from mast cells, leading to severe hypotension. The cause of the hypotension is peripheral vasodilation and sympathetic ganglionic blockade. Perhaps of even more concern to patients in respiratory failure is the bronchospasm with excessive bronchial and salivary secretions produced by the released histamine.

An alternative to using competitive neuromuscular blockers of the *d*-tubocurarine type is the use of succinylcholine. As mentioned above, succinylcholine differs from *d*-tubocurarine in its mechanism of action by causing persistent depolarization of the motor end-plate. Succinylcholine is administered intravenously and has a rapid onset of action (within 1 minute) and a short duration of action (approximately 5 minutes), largely because of its rapid hydrolysis by pseudocholinesterase in the plasma and the liver. Muscular relaxation of longer duration can be achieved by repeated injections or by continuous infusion. Prior to causing paralysis, transient muscle fasciculations occur, which may partially explain the muscle soreness that follows succinylcholine use. A smooth response has been reported for the infusion of a 0.1% solution at a rate of 2 to 3 mg/minute.

In approximately 1/3000 of the population, succinylcholine will be hydrolyzed at a reduced rate because of the presence of an atypical pseudocholinesterase. In these patients, prolonged muscular relaxation and apnea lasting several hours can occur. Succinylcholine apnea is a genetically transmitted predisposition that, if suspected, can be tested for by determining a dibucaine number. Another side effect of succinylcholine that has a familial component is malignant hyperthermia. In susceptible patients receiving halothane and succinylcholine, a severe rapid rise in temperature can occur, which may be fatal unless managed properly. Malignant hyperthermia should be treated by rapid cooling, inhalation of 100% oxygen, and control of the acidosis that is normally present.

Acute cardiovascular collapse may also follow intravenous succinylcholine administration. This is believed to be the result of potassium efflux from skeletal muscle during persistent depolarization. The resultant hyperkalemia may produce myocardial depression and ventricular arrhythmias.

A newer drug that appears to have certain definite advantages over *d*-tubocurarine and succinylcholine is pancuronium bromide. Its principal desirable features are its nearly complete absence of adverse cardiovascular effects and of the tendency to release histamine. Thus, it appears to be the drug of choice. For endotracheal intubation, intravenous injection of pancuronium will produce relaxation in 2 to 3 minutes, lasting up to 90 minutes.

RESPIRATORY DEPRESSANTS

A number of different classes of drugs have as an undesirable side effect the ability to depress respiration. This is of particular concern in patients who already have acute or chronic underlying pulmonary diseases (*e.g.*, asthma, chronic obstructive pulmonary disorders) or who are elderly with compromised hepatic and renal functions. Probably the greatest offenders as respiratory depressants are opiate and nonopiate analgesics and hypnotic-sedative drugs.

Opiates and Nonopiate Analgesics

Morphine has a direct, dose-related depressant effect on the brain stem respiratory centers. The mechanism involves a reduction in the sensitivity of the brain stem respiratory centers to CO_2. Its main effect is a decrease in respiratory rate, which diminishes respiratory volume and tidal exchange. Respiratory arrest is the principal cause of death in humans from morphine intoxication. Because morphine can cause tissues to release histamine, there is an added basis for avoiding the use of this narcotic in most asthmatics.

The most familiar of the nonopiates is meperidine. It possesses respiratory depressant effects equal to those of morphine, and can also depress neonatal breathing when given during parturition. Meperidine, therefore, offers no significant benefits over morphine as an analgesic for respiratory patients.

Fentanyl is a very potent analgesic that is used independently or as an adjunct for anesthesia induction. It is also a powerful respiratory depressant. In fact, fentanyl is considered to be a hazardous drug for patients with impaired respiratory function, and its use should be avoided in these individuals. Fentanyl use is also associated with delayed respiratory depression (lasting several hours) in patients recovering from anesthesia.

Pentazocine is a popular drug used for the treatment of moderate pain. Unfortunately, it can produce significant respiratory depression and should not be used in conjunction with other narcotics. Pentazocine use should be avoided in patients with asthma or other forms of respiratory distress.

Among the strong nonopiate analgesics, ethoheptazine and methotrimeprazine produce the least degree of respiratory depression. These would appear to be likely alternatives to the use of morphine or meperidine in respiratory patients.

Opiate Antagonists

Mechanisms of Action. The various effects produced by opiates are the result of stereospecific binding to a group of receptors, among which are the μ, κ, and σ receptors. The respiratory depression that is one of the undesirable side effects of opiate use is believed to be the result of binding of the opiate to the μ receptor in the brain. Structural analogs of morphine (the prototypic opiate) have been synthesized that have varying degrees of agonism, partial agonism, or antagonism for the various receptor types.

Naloxone. Naloxone is the drug closest to being a pure competitive antagonist, with no agonistic effect for any of the receptor types (Fig. 2–4). Naloxone is thought to have the highest affinity for μ receptors, with no intrinsic activity to produce respiratory depression. This important feature distinguishes naloxone from other obsolete antagonists such as

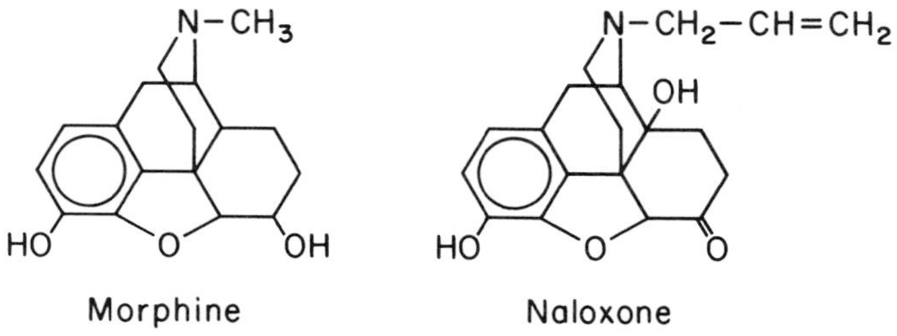

Morphine   Naloxone

Figure 2-4. Structural relationship of the prototypic opiate morphine to its antagonist, naloxone.

levallorphan and nalorphine, which can themselves cause respiratory depression.

Naloxone is the safest and most preferred drug for treating respiratory depression produced by known or suspected narcotic intoxication, including nonopiates such as meperidine. Naloxone also blocks the depressant effects of the endogenous opiate β-endorphin. Doses of naloxone on the order of 0.4 to 0.8 mg given parenterally produce an effect within several minutes that can last for 3 to 5 hours. Special preparations for use in neonates are also available.

Sedative-Hypnotics

These two types of psychotropic drugs are generally employed therapeutically for their calming effect as well as for the management of insomnia and for daytime sedation. Whether or not drugs in this category will exacerbate compromised respiratory function appears to depend on how judiciously they are used. It is generally agreed that sedative doses of secobarbital, pentobarbital, and cyclobarbital produce no significant depression of respiration. However, careless use in patients with chronic obstructive pulmonary diseases can cause respiratory failure. Ideally, their use should be avoided or minimized because of their central depressant effects. If a sedative-hypnotic does have to be used in a patient with asthma, for example, a short-acting agent with minimal respiratory depressive effects should be selected.

Because all barbiturates are respiratory depressants, it has been suggested that they not be used at all as hypnotics in respiratory patients. However, even though the neurogenic drive can be diminished by hypnotic doses, it is usually no more so than during sleep. Elimination of neurogenic drive requires three times the normal hypnotic dose. If an alternative to barbiturate use in a respiratory patient is deemed necessary, use of the substituted alcohols may be appropriate. For example, chloral betaine and triclofos sodium have little effect on respiration when given in therapeutic doses. These drugs have certain advantages over the parent drug chloral hydrate, which has been reported to be useful and safe as a sedative in asthmatics and as a hypnotic in patients with respiratory insufficiency. In addition, the benzodiazepine flurazepam can be used as a hypnotic, and produces less respiratory depression than the barbiturates.

Minor Tranquilizers

With the exception of flurazepam, benzodiazepines are primarily employed as minor tranquilizers for the treatment of various anxiety disorders. As a group they are less likely to cause respiratory depression than barbiturates, but have about the same effects as other sedative-hypnotics. Diazepam may be safer in patients with respiratory insufficiency, particularly when administered orally. The dicarbamates meprobamate and tybamate are also used as minor tranquilizers, and appear to have a potential for producing ventilatory depression similar to that of the benzodiazepines.

Hydroxazine is a tranquilizer that also possesses antihistaminic and bronchodilator (anticholinergic) properties. It is, therefore, a useful sedative-hypnotic or tranquilizer for anxious patients with bronchospastic diseases. It is a drug of choice for the preanesthesia preparation of patients with ventilatory inadequacy.

Major Tranquilizers and Antidepressants

A number of drugs are valuable because of their antipsychotic properties. Antipsychotic agents include the phenothiazines (*e.g.*, chlorpromazine), thioxanthanes (*e.g.*, chlorprothixene), butyrophenones (*e.g.*, haloperidol), dibenzodiazepines (*e.g.*, clozapine) and rauwolfia alkaloids (*e.g.*, reserpine). They are frequently used on respiratory care units to treat the severe stress-related psychoses that can develop. Fortunately, they have little tendency to produce respiratory depression, so they are of less concern when needed by patients with chronic obstructive airway diseases. Similarly, antidepressants such as the tricyclic compounds (*e.g.*, amitriptyline hydrochloride) do not depress respiration at usual doses and may, in fact, decrease bronchospasm (anticholinergics).

SELECTED REFERENCES

Borison, H. L.: Central respiratory depressants—narcotic analgesics. *In* Widdicombe, J. G., (ed.): Respiratory Pharmacology, Section 104, International Encyclopedia of Pharmacology and Therapeutics, Oxford, Pergamon Press, 1981, pp. 53–63.
Borison, H. L.: Central nervous respiratory depressants—anesthetics, hypnotics, sedatives and other respiratory depressants. *In* Widdicombe, J. G. (ed.): Respiratory Pharmacol-

ogy, Section 104, International Encyclopedia of Pharmacology and Therapeutics, Oxford, Pergamon Press, 1981, pp. 65–83.

Donahue, J.: Control of ventilation. *In* Gong, H., and Drage, C. (eds.): Norwalk, Appleton-Century-Crofts, 1980, pp. 95–104.

Gautier, H., and Vincent, J.: Muscle relaxants and breathing. *In* Widdicombe, J. G. (ed.): Respiratory Pharmacology, New York, Pergamon Press, 1981, pp. 335–342.

Gelb, A. W., Southhorn, P., and Rehder, K.: Effect of general anaesthesia on respiratory function. Lung, 1959:187, 1981.

Luce, J., Tyler, M., and Pierson, D.: Respiration and the anatomy of the respiratory system. *In* Luce, J., Tyler, M., and Pierson, D. (eds.): Intensive Respiratory Care, Philadelphia, W. B. Saunders, 1984, pp. 1–15.

Mueller, R., et al.: The neuropharmacology of respiratory control. Pharmacol. Rev., 34:255, 1982.

West, J. B.: Human physiology at extreme altitudes on Mount Everest. Science, 223:784, 1984.

CHAPTER 3

Nonrespiratory Lung Functions

UPTAKE AND METABOLISM OF VASOACTIVE SUBSTANCES

As mentioned previously, the lungs receive the cardiac output first, whereupon it is distributed within a vast network of pulmonary vessels. The blood that traverses the alveolar-capillary area is exposed to high P_{O_2} and low P_{CO_2} in the alveolar air, leading to a net exchange of CO_2 for O_2. It is now known that this is not the only important physiologic function carried out in this particular region.

It is clear that the lung can also take up, accumulate, and metabolize a number of endogenous and exogenous substances. Among the endogenous substances that have been shown to be significantly inactivated by the lungs of all animals studied to date are biogenic amines (norepinephrine and 5-hydroxytryptamine), prostaglandins, polypeptides, and nucleotides.

The specificity of the lung for metabolizing substances *in vivo* is a result of its structural organization, particularly in regard to functions associated with the capillary endothelial cell. This can be demonstrated by homogenizing lung tissue. Homogenization destroys this compartmentalization and results in the liberation of enzymes, which show little substrate discrimination once access to the enzymes is gained.

Biogenic Amines

One of the first reports dealing with the pulmonary removal of an endogenous substance from the blood involved the uptake of norepinephrine by an isolated dog lung. In this study, it was found that 96% of the administered catecholamine was removed within a 30-minute period. Since then the lungs of several other species, including the cat, the rabbit, the rat, and the human have been shown to have this same ability to remove norepinephrine.

More recent studies using isolated rat lung preparations indicate that the uptake of norepinephrine by the lung occurs in endothelial cells, and is a carrier-mediated saturable process with high affinity. This type of uptake process requires energy, and is temperature-sensitive and sodium-dependent. Following uptake, norepinephrine is quickly metabolized; it has been reported that 80% can be metabolized during a 5-minute infusion. Metabolism is carried out primarily by catechol-O-methyltransferase (COMT) and monoamine oxidase (MAO). However, the active transport of norepinephrine is the rate-limiting step in overall removal, not enzyme activity.

The pulmonary uptake system for norepinephrine appears to be quite similar to the reuptake mechanism for norepinephrine that is found in neuronal tissue. The major difference is that, following reuptake in a nerve terminal, norepinephrine is not metabolized but is rebound for further release. Other extraneuronal sites of norepinephrine uptake, such as the heart, are not as similar. A comparison of some norepinephrine uptake criteria in pulmonary, neuronal, and extraneuronal (heart) tissue is shown in Table 3–1.

In addition to high affinity, the norepinephrine uptake process is quite specific. For example, there is negligible or no pulmonary uptake of close structural analogs, such as epinephrine, isoproterenol, L-dopa, and dopamine. Other aromatic lipophilic basic amines such as propranolol, lidocaine, imipramine, amphetamine, methadone, and chlorcyclizine can accumulate in the lung but do so by passive diffusion. Because they are slowly released in their original forms, the lung can serve as a reservoir for these drugs.

Another amine that has been extensively studied is serotonin (5-hydroxytryptamine; 5-HT). Studies in anesthetized animals and in isolated lung preparations have shown that, depending on the species used, up to 98% of an infusion of 5-HT can be removed by endothelial cells in a single passage through the pulmonary circulation. In fact, it is possible that the lung actually contributes more to the clearance of 5-HT from the blood than does the liver. Analysis of lung perfusates indicate that this rapid removal is associated with almost total conversion of 5-HT to 5-hydroxyindoleacetic acid catalyzed by monoamine oxidase A. Formation

Table 3–1. Comparison of Norepinephrine Uptake Systems

Characteristic	Pulmonary	Neuronal	Extraneuronal
Metabolized by MAO and COMT	+	−	+
Sodium-dependent	+	+	+ −
Temperature-dependent	+	+	+
Inhibited by ouabain	+	+	−
Inhibited by cocaine	+	+	−
Inhibited by tricyclic antidepressants	+	+	−
Michaelis constant (K_m)	1–2.4×10^{-6} M	6.6×10^{-7} M	2.5×10^{-4} M

of the deaminated metabolite occurs within minutes, with conversion of more than 90% of the 5-HT taken up. The rate-limiting step in this process is uptake, which has a K_m* of approximately 5 μM.

Experiments in isolated lungs of the rabbit and the rat indicate that the pulmonary process for uptake of 5-HT is similar to that of norepinephrine in that it requires energy, is temperature- and sodium-dependent, and is saturable. In addition, the uptake of 5-HT in the lung is also inhibited by ouabain, cocaine, and tricyclic antidepressants such as imipramine.

Despite the similarities, however, 5-HT and norepinephrine are undoubtedly taken up by different sites, because the presence of great excesses of norepinephrine do not significantly reduce 5-HT uptake. In addition, 5-HT transport sites appear to be evenly distributed throughout the vasculature, whereas norepinephrine transport may occur primarily in pre- and postcapillary vessels.

Because uptake of 5-HT and norepinephrine is dependent on endothelial surface area, any reduction will be reflected in the pulmonary venous concentration. Such measurements are presently being carried out in humans to assess lung microvascular status. The significance of pulmonary clearance of 5-HT can be appreciated, because a 5% decrease has been calculated to result in a doubling of the amine concentration surviving transpulmonary transit.

Prostaglandins

Prostaglandins (PGs) are fatty acids of the prostanoid family with great biologic significance because of their ubiquity, high potency, and diversity of effects. They were originally discovered during the 1930s in studies dealing with the contractile effect of human seminal plasma on uterine smooth muscle strips. Purification was eventually carried out using sheep prostate glands—hence the name. Chemically, PGs are classified as prostanoic acid derivatives, which vary according to the substituents on the cyclopentane ring (*e.g.*, E or F type) and the number of double bonds in the side chains (subscript). These characteristics are the basis for PG nomenclature (Fig. 3–1).

Of all the organs that have been studied, the lungs are among the most active in forming PGs. Parenchymal tissue appears to contain primarily $PGF_{2\alpha}$, while PGE_2 is mainly associated with bronchial walls. The sites of PG synthesis in the lung include endothelial cells, alveolar macrophages, fibroblasts, and type II cells. These cells are extremely rich in a complex of cyclo-oxygenase enzymes known collectively as prosta-

---

*Drug concentration at one-half maximum velocity.

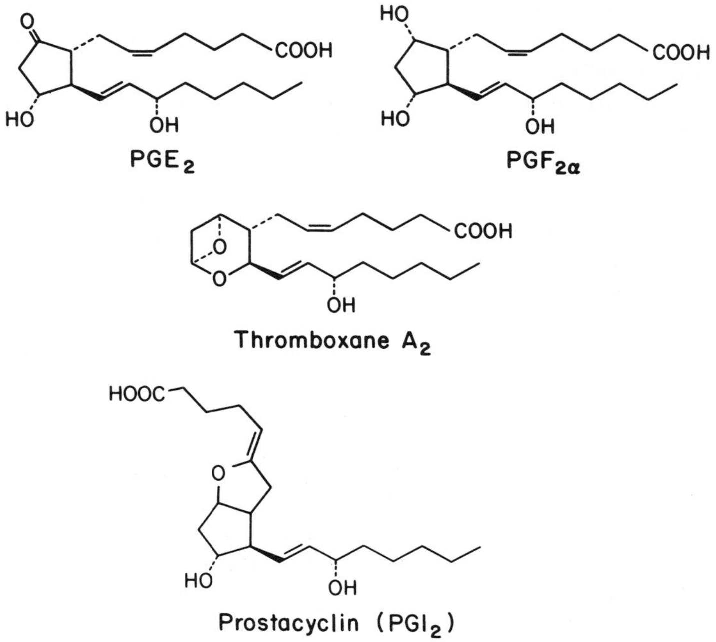

PGE_2

$PGF_{2\alpha}$

Thromboxane A_2

Prostacyclin (PGI_2)

Figure 3–1. Comparison of the chemical structures of various prostanoids.

glandin synthetase. A summary of pharmacologic and physiologic actions of PGs and related compounds is shown in Table 3-2.

The biosynthetic pathway for PGs, as well as for the related prostanoids leukotrienes, prostacyclins, and thromboxanes, is shown in Figure 3-2. Because PGs are not stored, synthesis is equivalent to release. The rate-limiting enzyme in PG synthesis is phospholipase A_2, which frees arachidonic acid from phospholipid stores in cellular membranes. Phospholipase A_2 can be activated by physical, hormonal, or chemical factors. Largely on the basis of experiments performed with guinea pigs, the principal PGs formed in the lungs appear to be PGE_2, $PGF_{2\alpha}$, and PGD_2 (in descending order).

In addition to being a rich source of PGs, the lung is also a principal source of PG-catabolizing enzymes. Available evidence strongly indicates that the pulmonary circulation is, in fact, the major site of metabolism of bloodborne PGs. In ascending order, the pulmonary removal of PGs is PGA, PGF, and PGE. Although PGA is little affected, PGE and PGF are almost completely removed during a single passage through the pulmonary circulation. In one passage through the lung, for example, inactivation of exogenous PGEs is 95% complete. Depending on species and technique, the K_m of the pulmonary removal system for PGE is 5 to 9 μM. The relative failure of PGA to be inactivated appears to be the result of the selectivity of the capillary endothelial cell transport system.

Following the uptake of prostaglandins into endothelial cells by a carrier-mediated transport system, a rapid two-stage metabolism is believed to take place. This sequence involves dehydrogenase and reductase enzymes. The result is the formation of 15-keto-13,14-dihydro-PGs. Leukotrienes are also inactivated by the lungs, whereas prostacyclin (PCI_2) is not. The net effect of the lung's variable metabolism of prostaglandins is that PGE_2, $PGF_{2\alpha}$, and leukotrienes are restricted to "local" hormonal roles. For example, PGE_2 has a half-life of less than 30 seconds in the peripheral circulation, and normal plasma concentrations are less than 12 pg/ml. On the other hand, PGA_2 and prostacyclin have a greater "systemic" effect, because they are metabolized to a smaller extent by the lung. In fact, the lung has been suggested as having an endocrine function by releasing prostacyclin. Prostacyclin's two main properties are relaxation of arteries and prevention of platelet aggregation. These are currently the subject of intensive study.

Because the lung is an important site for prostaglandin inactivation, the question of the effect that an injured lung has on the pharmacodynamics of systemic prostaglandins may be important. It has been found that ozone, cigarette smoke, bleomycin, monocrotaline, paraquat, and cardiopulmonary bypass can suppress the pulmonary inactivation of PGs. However, the clinical significance of these observations is unknown.

Probably the greatest significance of prostaglandins in the lung is related to their effects on vascular and respiratory smooth muscles. For example, $PGF_{2\alpha}$ and its 15-keto metabolite are both bronchoconstrictors and appear to play a role in the development of asthma, allergic reactions, and inflammation. Studies indicate that blood levels of $PGF_{2\alpha}$ are higher in patients with asthma than in healthy control subjects. Asthmatics are also substantially more sensitive to $PGF_{2\alpha}$. In one study of asthmatic patients, for example, $PGF_{2\alpha}$ was about 10,000 times more active than in normal subjects. In comparison, asthmatics are about ten times more sensitive to histamine. Because of the sensitivity of asthmatics to $PGF_{2\alpha}$, a history of bronchial asthma is now recognized as a relative contraindication for the use of $PGF_{2\alpha}$ to induce therapeutic abortion.

On the other hand, bronchial smooth muscle is relaxed by PGE. PGE_1 is approximately 70 times more potent than isoproterenol in producing bronchodilation, with a duration comparable to that of the catecholamines. PGE can also antagonize the effect of bronchospasmogens such as histamine and 5-HT. Unfortunately, clinical trials to date with aerosol-administered PGEs indicate that their usefulness may be limited by their irritant actions on the respiratory tract that produce coughing and soreness. Under normal physiologic circumstances, PGE and β-adrenergic agonists probably play an antagonistic role to $PGF_{2\alpha}$ in regulating respiratory airway smooth muscle patency.

Leukotrienes are also receiving a great deal of attention at present because of their putative role in allergic reactions such as asthma. In

Table 3–2. Local and Systemic Effects of Pulmonary Arachidonic Acid Metabolites*

Metabolite	Effect on Bronchial Smooth Muscle	Effect on Pulmonary Vascular Smooth Muscle	Systemic Effects	Important Characteristics
PGE_2	Dilation	Usually vasodilation	Vasodilation; reduces mucus secretion and platelet aggregation	Rapidly inactivated by lung endothelium; inhibits histamine release from basophils; probably arises from lung parenchyma
$PGF_{2\alpha}$	Constriction	Constriction	Variable vasoconstriction; increases mucus secretion; antagonizes thromboxane A_2–induced platelet aggregation	Rapidly inactivated by lung endothelium; probably arises from bronchial smooth muscle
PGD_2	Constriction	Constriction	Decreases mucus secretion; enhances histamine release from basophils; chemotactic for eosinophils	Mast cell is probably a major source
Prostacyclin (PGI_2)	Dilation	Dilation	Vasodilation; inhibits platelet aggregation; increases mucus secretion; inhibits histamine release from basophils	Synthesized by endothelial cells; short-lived, but not primarily metabolized by lung endothelium; inhibits leukocyte aggregation

Thromboxane (TxA$_2$)	Constriction	Constriction	Increases platelet aggregation and leukocyte adhesiveness; inhibits release of leukotrienes	Found in platelets; very active and short-lived; component of rabbit aorta contracting substance (RCS); metabolized to inactive TxB$_2$
Leukotrienes (LTs)	Constriction (LTB$_4$ less active than LTC$_4$, LTD$_4$ and LTE$_4$)	Constriction by LTC$_4$ and LTD$_4$; dilation by LTE$_4$	Increased capillary permeability and mucus release; decreased tracheal mucus velocity; release of TxA$_2$ and prostaglandins from lung; chemotactic for leukocytes	LTC$_4$, LTD$_4$, and LTE$_4$ are components of slow-reacting substance of anaphylaxis (SRS-A); some effects are mediated by prostaglandins; formed in mast cells and others
Hydroxyeicosatetraenoic acids (HETEs)			Enhance release of histamine from mast cells and basophils; enhance phagocytic function of polymorphs; chemotactic for leukocytes; increase mucus secretion	Function as proinflammatory factors

*Some of these effects may vary according to species, dosage, route of administration, and the experimental design used.

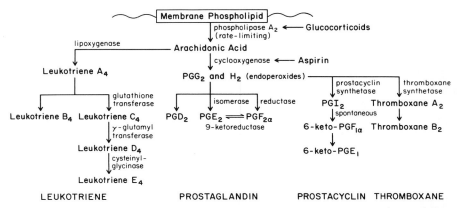

Figure 3–2. Biosynthetic pathway for the formation of several members of the prostanoid family.

humans, leukotrienes are potent bronchoconstrictive agents, and may significantly contribute to the edema and mucous hypersecretion also observed in asthma. On a weight-for-weight basis, leukotrienes C_4 and D_4 are at least 1000 times more potent than histamine in causing contraction of isolated human bronchi. It is now known that the slow reacting substance of anaphylaxis (SRS-A), first reported in 1938, is a mixture of leukotrienes C_4, D_4, and E_4, and that their effects are mediated by separate receptors. Leukotriene D_4 appears to exert its bronchoconstrictive actions, by a direct pathway and by an indirect, thromboxane-dependent pathway, depending on its mode of administration. Intravenous administration elicits bronchoconstriction by both indirect and direct mechanisms, whereas aerosol administration does so only by the direct pathway. Leukotriene B_4 is also an extremely potent chemotactic and chemokinetic agent that can elicit a rapid accumulation of eosinophils and a delayed accumulation of neutrophils. It has been found to cause contraction of various smooth muscles, to release lysosomal enzymes, and to increase cyclic nucleotide levels. These biologic activities strongly suggest an important role for leukotriene B_4 in allergic and inflammatory states.

Some drugs are known to inhibit PG synthesis, including meclofenamic acid, niflumic acid, indomethacin, mefenamic acid, flufenamic acid, naproxen, phenylbutazone, aspirin, and ibuprofen. These nonsteroidal anti-inflammatory agents act by inhibiting the cyclooxygenase step and by the subsequent participation of PGs in pain, fever, and inflammation. These drugs will also prevent the formation of thromboxanes.

Steroidal anti-inflammatory drugs such as glucocorticoids also interfere with PG formation but apparently do so by blocking arachidonic acid release. This blockade is believed to be the result of stimulating the formation of an inhibitor (lipomodulin) of phospholipase A_2. By inhibiting the release of arachidonic acid, steroids prevent formation of not only

PGs and thromboxanes but also of leukotrienes. The latter effect may be responsible for some of the therapeutic differences in the anti-inflammatory properties of steroids that are not shared by aspirin-type drugs.

Structural analogs of PGs have also been found that inhibit the dehydrogenase enzyme. Studies are presently being done to develop the following: drugs that will specifically inhibit $PGF_{2\alpha}$ formation in the lung while not effecting PGE synthesis; new analogs with longer duration of action and less irritating properties; new delivery systems for improved PGE introduction into the lung; end-organ antagonists to $PGF_{2\alpha}$ and leukotrienes; and inhibitors of leukotriene release.

Polypeptides

Electron photomicroscopic examination of the surface of pulmonary endothelial cells reveals a series of membrane-covered indentations (caveolae). Residing on the luminal side of the membrane are clusters of a dipeptidylcarboxypeptidase called angiotensin-converting enzyme (ACE). Each endothelial cell contains approximately 1,000,000 molecules of ACE. Although ACE is distributed throughout the body, the lungs contain the greatest total amount. This enzyme is responsible for the activation of the decapeptide angiotensin I to the pressor octapeptide angiotensin II, as well as the inactivation of the hypotensive agent bradykinin (Fig. 3–3). Bradykinin is the preferred substrate for the enzyme, with K_m values ranging from 20- to 100-fold less than for angiotensin I. The lung, therefore, has the potential to play an important physiologic role in hemodynamic regulation. However, few clinical or clinically related studies have been performed to examine the pathophysiologic consequences of this processing.

Because of its role in the conversion of angiotensin I to angiotensin II, ACE is a terminal component of the renin-angiotensin system. Acti-

$H_2N-Asp-Arg-Val-Tyr-Ile-His-Pro-Phe-His-Leu-COOH$ **Angiotensin I**

↓   ↑ ACE

$H_2N-Asp-Arg-Val-Tyr-Ile-His-Pro-Phe-COOH$ **Angiotensin II**

$H_2N-Arg-Pro-Pro-Gly-Phe-Ser-Pro-Phe-Arg-COOH$ **Bradykinin**

↓   ↑ ACE

$H_2N-Arg-Pro-Pro-Gly-Phe-Ser-Pro-COOH$ **Metabolite**

Figure 3–3. Mechanism of action of angiotensin-converting enzyme (ACE) in activating angiotensin and inactivating bradykinin.

vation of this pathway occurs via the formation of angiotensin I from angiotensinogen by renin. This, in effect, produces more substrate for pulmonary ACE and, concomitantly, a corresponding increase in blood pressure. Renin can be released from the kidney by factors such as low blood volume, low renal perfusion pressure, and low plasma sodium concentration.

Obviously, if ACE could be inhibited, it might be expected that peripheral resistance would be lowered by decreasing the formation of angiotensin II and by prolonging the action of bradykinin. This has, in fact, been found to be the case in studies initially carried out with pit viper venoms. These venoms were found to contain a family of peptides with 5 to 13 amino acid residues that could inhibit lung ACE. These observations have provided a foundation for the development of a relatively new class of antihypertensive agents. However, because peptides in general are inactivated when given orally, resistant carboxyalkanoyl or mercaptoalkanoyl peptide derivatives had to be developed. One of these, D-3-mercapto-methylpropanoyl-L-proline (captopril) is now routinely used clinically for the treatment of certain forms of hypertension (Fig. 3–4).

Angiotensin I and bradykinin have been the most intensively studied polypeptides metabolized by the lung. However, it now appears that they are not the only peptides that can interact with ACE. Recent studies indicate that the opioid peptides β-endorphin, methionine enkephalin, and leucine enkephalin, as well as adrenocorticotropic hormone and substance P, can also compete for the enzyme. Substrate specificity does exist, though, because peptides such as oxytocin, vasopressin, and vasoactive intestinal peptide (VIP) do not appear to be metabolized by the enzyme. These observations suggest that the pulmonary role(s) of ACE may be more complex and far-reaching than previously thought.

Nucleotides

Over 30 years ago it was demonstrated that the lung can remove adenosine triphosphate (ATP) from the pulmonary arterial circulation. This removal process has since been shown to be the result of phosphate esterases that are also located in caveolae on endothelial cells. The lung can also inactivate adenosine monophosphate and diphosphate (AMP and ADP), potent platelet-aggregating agents. Unfortunately, there has been relatively little follow-up work done on these observations. Therefore, the physiologic significance of the lung's ability to metabolize adenine nucleotides is still unclear.

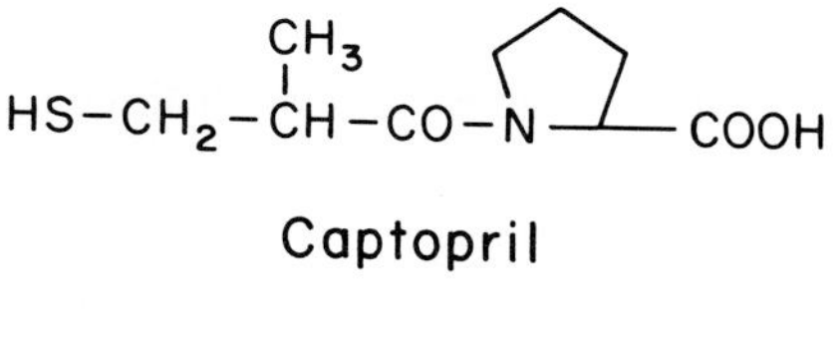

$$HS-CH_2-\overset{\overset{\textstyle CH_3}{|}}{CH}-CO-N \diagup\!\!\!\diagdown\!\!- COOH$$

Captopril

Figure 3–4. Structure of the antihypertensive drug captopril, an inhibitor of ACE.

One intriguing possibility has been suggested, though. This involves adenosine, a product of ATP metabolism. Among its pharmacologic effects are vasodilation, constriction of the bronchial tree, and antiplatelet aggregation. The suggestion has been made that, under conditions of lung injury, adenine nucleotides may be released from pulmonary tissue and metabolized to adenosine, which then acts as a local vasodilator and antithrombotic factor. Interestingly, the compound dipyridamole, which has antithrombotic effects, can prevent the uptake of adenosine by endothelial cells. Additional work will have to be done to clarify these hypothetic roles as well as to define more clearly the significance of pulmonary nucleotide uptake in general.

Effect of Lung Damage on Clearance of Endogenous Substances

In view of the fact that the lung can remove and metabolize a number of circulating endogenous agents, measurements of these pharmacokinetic functions could conceivably provide a useful index for assessment of pulmonary microvascular injury. During the last 10 years, several laboratories have been studying this process. Most of these studies have dealt with 5-HT clearance although other systems, such as those involving the PGs and angiotensin, are receiving increased attention.

Among the pneumotoxins that have been investigated as models are hyperbaric oxygen, anoxia, halothane, nitrous dioxide, paraquat, and chlorphentermine. In animal studies, hyperbaric oxygen has been shown to decrease pulmonary clearance of 5-HT by inhibiting its transport into the endothelial cells. This inhibitory effect by oxygen is reversible, and may involve the local generation of toxic superoxide anions. Hyperbaric oxygen has also been reported to decrease pulmonary clearance of norepinephrine and PGE_2. The effect of hyperbaric oxygen on PG clearance appears to be on PG dehydrogenase (metabolism) rather than on transport. Anoxia has been reported to decrease the activity of ACE in intact lungs and in cultured endothelial cells. The anesthetic gas halothane has been reported to inhibit the metabolism of norepinephrine in intact dog lungs and in perfused rabbit lung. Studies in the perfused rat lung indicate that halothane inhibits 5-HT metabolism by reducing its uptake.

It is interesting to note that the effect of acute hyperbaric oxygen on 5-HT transport (presumably at the membrane) occurs prior to that on prostaglandin metabolism (intracellular), suggesting that the former parameter is a more responsive index of endothelial cell damage. Nitrous dioxide has also been reported to inhibit pulmonary PG metabolism. This evidence strongly suggests that endothelial cells are probably affected more than is generally recognized.

In addition to the gases mentioned above, systemically transported lung toxicants can also alter amine uptake. The herbicide paraquat, when administered parenterally to rats, significantly reduces 5-HT clearance by the lung. The decrease in 5-HT removal is the result of an impairment of its carrier-mediated transport into the endothelial cells. Significantly, the depression of 5-HT uptake by rat lung exposed to paraquat occurs prior to the appearance of morphologic changes (24 hours). Similar results have been obtained with the pneumotoxins α-napthylthiourea, bleomycin, and monocrotaline. These results suggest that measurement of 5-HT uptake, norepinephrine uptake, or the uptake of both might serve as an early indicator of microvascular injury in the lung.

Chlorphentermine is a drug that has been used for weight reduction and implicated in the development of pulmonary hypertension. Recent studies indicate that chlorphentermine reduces pulmonary clearance of 5-HT by inhibiting its metabolism and its uptake (see Hypertension, below).

Morpholine is another example of how chemical exposure might alter pulmonary clearance of a drug. This chemical is an industrial solvent used in the manufacture of resins, waxes, and dyes. Exposure of rabbits to morpholine vapor results in pulmonary damage, a decrease in alveolar macrophage enzyme activity, and reduced pulmonary uptake of imipramine (see below: Uptake and Accumulation of Basic Amines: Mechanisms). Apparently, morpholine injures alveolar macrophages, which normally can take up a certain proportion of imipramine.

The possibility is raised, therefore, that industrial exposure to noxious vapors or chemicals could have an effect on the clearance of both endogenous amines and drugs by the lung. In the same context, several studies using animal lungs indicate that gaseous anesthetics such as halothane and nitrous oxide can reduce the inactivation of 5-HT and norepinephrine. This observation has yet to be confirmed in humans, however.

UPTAKE AND ACCUMULATION OF BASIC AMINES

Mechanisms

As described above, it is quite clear that the lung can accumulate several endogenous compounds. This section will review the equally important observation that exogenous pharmacologic and toxicologic agents can also be accumulated by the lung. Although these studies have been carried out in experimental animals such as the rat, guinea pig, dog, rabbit, and monkey, there is no reason not to expect that similarly high lung-to-blood ratios can occur in the human. Some of the more common drugs and toxicants reported to concentrate in animal lungs are listed in Table 3–3.

Analysis of these chemicals indicates one predominating feature that is generally shared: that is, they tend to be highly lipophilic amines with a pK_a higher than 8. There must be other important characteristics as well,

Table 3–3. Examples of Drugs and Toxicants Reported to Accumulate in the Lung

β-*Adrenergic Blocking Agents* Propranolol	***Antimalarials*** Chloroquine Primaquine
Amphetamines Amphetamine β-Monofluoramphetamine β,β-Difluoramphetamine Chloramphetamine	***Antipsychotics*** Fluphenazine Clozapine
	Furans 4-Ipomeanol 3-Methylfuran 2-(*N*-ethylcarbamoylhydroxymethyl)furan
Analgesics and Narcotics Methadone Morphine Δ^9-Tetrahydrocannabinol	
	Herbicides and Pesticides Paraquat Nicotine
Anorectic Drugs Chlorphentermine Phentermine	***Local Anesthetic*** Lidocaine
Antibiotic Nitrofurantoin	***Substituted Ureas*** Thiourea α-Naphthylthiourea
Antidepressants (Tricyclic) Imipramine Desimipramine	
Antihistamines Cyclizine Chlorcyclizine Diphenhydramine Tripelennamine	

however, because kinetic studies of several drugs clearly indicate that mechanisms of uptake, accumulation, and retention can vary. Nevertheless, possession of this chemical feature by a drug or toxin represents a strong predictive probability that the molecule will tend to accumulate in the lung.

The two most fundamental ways in which a drug or toxicant can accumulate in the lung are by active uptake (5-HT) or by decreased release. Imipramine is an example of the latter mechanism. Like most basic amines, imipramine seems to accumulate in the lung, primarily by diffusing in and being bound. Binding studies indicate that several efflux pools are formed because of varying degrees of reversible associations. This multicomponent binding system is composed of saturable and nonsaturable sites with long and short half-lives, respectively. The nature of the binding sites are unknown, but is believed to include alveolar surfactant phospholipids and macrophages.

Drugs such as amphetamine that resemble endogenous catecholamines appear to be taken up both by diffusion and by a carrier-mediated pulmonary transport system, which is probably identical to that described previously for catecholamines. They do not appear to form persistent pools in the lung.

Phospholipidosis

Because certain types of chemicals can accumulate in the lung, it is not surprising that a pattern of corresponding pneumotoxicity is beginning to emerge. One type of lung response that has been studied in this regard is phospholipidosis. Drug-induced phospholipidosis is based on the formation of a drug-phospholipid complex that cannot be degraded. Alveolar macrophages phagocytize the indigestible phospholipid and become "foam" cells. A representative list of chemicals that have been reported to produce lung phospholipidosis is shown in Table 3–4. Note the similarity between this list and the drugs and toxicants shown in Table 3–3 that can accumulate in the lungs.

Using the anorectic chlorphentermine as a model, it has been shown that chronic administration for several weeks results in a tissue-to-blood ratio several-fold greater in the lung than in the liver. An accumulation of chlorphentermine in the lung is the result of reversible binding to polar lipids by electrostatic and hydrophobic bonds. Accumulation of the phospholipid appears to occur as a result of decreased degradation of the drug-lipid complex by catabolic phospholipases. Significantly, chlorphentermine has been found to inhibit phospholipases A and C. Reduction of chlorphentermine accumulation in the lung has been reported in rats

---

Table 3–4. Chemicals Associated with Pulmonary Phospholipidosis

Antidepressants
  Iprindole
  Amitriptyline
  1-Choloramitriptyline
  1-Chloro-10,11-dehydroamitriptyline
  Noxiptyline
  Imipramine
  Clomipramine

Anorectics
  Chlorphentermine
  Fenfluramine
  cis-7-Fluoro-1-phenyl-3-isochromanmethylamine

Antimalarials
  Chloroquine
  4-Cyano-5-chlorophenylamidinourea

Cholesterol Biosynthesis Inhibitors
  Triparanol
  trans,1-4-*bis*-(chlorobenzylaminomethyl)cyclohexane
  Azacosterol

Neuroleptics
  Chlorpromazine
  Thioridazine

Miscellaneous
  4,4'-Diethylethoxyhexestrol
  2-*N*-Methylpiperazinomethyl-1,3-diazafluoroanethen-1-oxide

---

treated with phenobarbital; apparently the barbiturate increases chlorphentermine urinary excretion rather than metabolism.

The phospholipid found is distributed in the form of lamellated inclusion bodies between alveolar epithelial type I cells, vascular endothelial cells, smooth muscle cells, bronchiolar epithelium, and alveolar macrophages. Alveolar macrophages are the most susceptible to phospholipid accumulation, because they tend to store excess phospholipid. Type II alveolar epithelial cells seem to be resistant to phospholipid accumulation, because they apparently can secrete the lipid micelles into the alveolar space. However, electron photomicrographic analysis indicates morphologic change in type II cell mitochondria that is associated with an uncoupling of oxidative phosphorylation.

Hypertension

In addition to accumulating in the lung and causing a disturbance in lung phospholipid biochemistry, the process of accumulation can have other clinical implications. In Europe during 1967 and 1968, for example, there occurred a rapid increase in the incidence of primary vascular hypertension. Follow-up studies revealed that an anorectic drug called aminorex was responsible. The apparent mechanism was related to aminorex inhibiting 5-HT clearance from the lung, leading to pulmonary hypertension. Some tricyclic antidepressants have also been reported to produce cardiovascular toxicity. It is conceivable that reduced 5-HT clearance might also play a role in these cases.

Thus, the fact that the lung can selectively remove certain basic amines from the circulatory system has several important implications. First, this feature could be advantageous in designing drugs for the specific treatment of pulmonary disease (conversely, a toxicant that is a basic amine would be predicted to have the lung as a target organ). Second, the pharmaco- and toxicodynamics of a substance could be altered because of its sequestration and subsequent inactivation in the lung.

XENOBIOTIC METABOLISM

Basic Characteristics

To deal with foreign lipid-soluble molecules that can cross cell membranes, the body has developed a number of highly effective enzyme systems, which generally biotransform these xenobiotics into more polar and less lipid-soluble metabolites. These polar metabolites are necessarily more rapidly eliminated from the body than their lipid-soluble counterparts, because they will be reabsorbed to a lesser degree from the kidney and may, in fact, be more actively secreted by this organ.

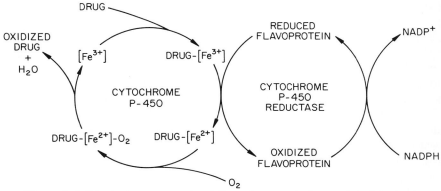

Figure 3–5. Principal components of the microsomal drug-metabolizing enzyme system.

The liver is the principal organ involved in xenobiotic metabolism. However, the lung possesses the second highest relative level of monooxygenase activity (10 to 20% that of liver). The term "monooxygenase" (also referred to as mixed function oxygenase) denotes a system of enzymes that insert oxygen into a foreign molecule. The pulmonary system for the oxidative metabolism of xenobiotics is quite similar to that of the liver. Subcellular localization is concentrated in the microsomal fraction, requires NADPH and O_2, and uses the enzymes NADPH-cytochrome c reductase and cytochrome P450 (a hemoprotein with maximal spectral absorbance at 450 nm). Like the hepatic system, the pulmonary system contains more than one form of P450 but at lower concentrations.

A schematic representation of the major components of the pulmonary microsomal drug-metabolizing enzyme system is shown in Figure 3–5. Enzyme assays of microsomal fractions and lung homogenates, as well as histochemical methods, indicate that some mixed function oxidase activity is present in alveolar macrophages as well as in alveolar and bronchiolar epithelial cells. However, in the lung, the Clara and type II cells appear to be the major sites of cytochrome P_{450}-dependent monooxygenase activity.

It has been discovered recently that the nasal mucosa of rodents also contains cytochrome P_{450}-dependent monooxygenases. These enzymes have been shown to metabolize compounds such as nasal decongestants, essences, solvents, air pollutants, nicotine, and cocaine to formaldehyde via N-demethylation. Perhaps the generation of formaldehyde in this area is related to the nasal mucosal irritation, olfaction variability, and carcinogenic characteristics associated with these chemicals. Furthermore, studies also indicate that mucosal damage produced by halogenated hydrocarbons (*e.g.*, chlorobenzene) is the result of local metabolism to toxic metabolites.

In addition to mixed function oxidase enzymes, there are other enzymes that can increase water solubility of a xenobiotic and enhance urinary or biliary excretion by attaching a small endogenous compound. These are conjugation enzymes such as glucuronyltransferase, sulfotransferase, glutathione S-aryltransferase, and N-acetyltransferase. All four of these enzymes have been found in the lung. Except for acetyltransferase, the activities of these enzymes are also much lower in the lung as compared to their activities in the liver. Despite the relative inferiority of the lung to the liver in metabolizing foreign substances, the lung nevertheless can biotransform a wide range of substances (Table 3–5).

Certain compounds are known to induce drug-metabolizing enzymes in the liver (increase *de novo* synthesis). These include phenobarbital, polyclic hydrocarbons (3-methylcholanthrene and benzo[*a*]pyrene), and certain steroids. Studies comparing the inducibility of drug-metabolizing enzymes in the liver and lung indicate that phenobarbital is generally less effective in the lung, whereas 3-methylcholanthrine and benzo[*a*]pyrene are more potent inducers of cytochrome P_{450} for the lung. The latter effect appears to be related to the formation of carcinogenic metabolites in the lung. Specific enzyme induction can occur in the lung, because 3-methylcholanthrene increases the metabolism of Δ^9-tetrahydrocannabinol in the lung but not in the liver.

As mentioned above, the process of biotransformation, whether it occurs in the liver or the lung, usually results in diminished activity. There are, however, certain situations in which metabolic alteration of a molecule in the lung can result in a metabolite with greater toxic potency rather than less (see below).

Formation of Active Intermediates

Biotransformation of a foreign molecule, in the liver or in the lung, generally results in a metabolite with less biologic activity and a more rapid rate of elimination from the body. Occurring less frequently are situations in which the metabolite that is formed from oxidative metabolism is actually more chemically reactive and more difficult to inactivate (whether toxin or drug). Carcinogens such as 3-methylcholanthrene and

Table 3–5. Representative Examples of Chemicals Metabolized by the Lung

Pesticides	*Narcotic Analgesics*	*Aromatic Hydrocarbons*
Aldrin	Methadone	Benzo[*a*]pyrene
Parathion	Mescaline	Benzo[*a*]pyrene-4,5-oxide
Nicotine	Δ^9-Tetrahydrocannabinol	
α-Naphthol		
Bronchodilators	*Miscellaneous*	
Dibuterol	Testosterone	
Terbutaline	Propranolol	
	Pentobarbital	

benzo[a]pyrene, for example, are not considered to be carcinogenic themselves, but rather their respective highly reactive metabolites are.

The mechanism(s) whereby active intermediates produce cell damage has been intensively studied during the last 10 years. One of the important discoveries made during this period is that certain chemically reactive metabolites generated *in vivo* can covalently bind by alkylation, acylation, or arylation to major cell components such as nucleic acids, protein, or lipids. This tight binding has been associated with tissue injury induced by numerous chemicals (*e.g.*, acetaminophen, furosemide, chloramphenicol) in various organs (*e.g.*, liver, kidney, bone marrow).

Active Intermediate Interaction in the Lung

Various pneumotoxins have also been shown to have their toxicity associated with the formation of reactive electrophiles; the following group of substances has been reported to bind covalently to lung or to respiratory tract macromolecules: bromobenzene; chlorobenzene; carbon tetrachloride; 2-(N-ethylcarbamoylhydroxymethyl) furan; 4-ipomeanol; 3-methylfuran; α-napthylthiourea; nitrofurantoin; pyrrolizidine alkaloids; thiourea; naphthalene; 2-methylnapthalene; 3-methylindole; and butylated hydroxytoluene. Covalent binding to tissue macromolecules is a characteristic of the members of this group of chemicals. Agents such as thiourea (and its analogs) and the sweet potato toxin 4-ipomeanol have been extensively studied in animal models. Although the exact relationship of covalent binding to tissue damage is unknown, it is recognized that reduced glutathione (GSH) can be important in modulating toxicity. In this capacity, GSH is believed to function as an intracellular nucleophile against electrophilic metabolites.

Apparently GSH can conjugate some of these highly reactive intermediates, thereby protecting critical cellular constituents against oxidative damage. This conjugation is catalyzed by a group of cytosolic glutathione S-transferase isoenzymes. In the process, intracellular levels of GSH will decrease. Figure 3–6 presents an example of this effect following the administration of the pulmonary edematogenic agent thiourea to the rat. If the GSH content can be exhausted, then excess intermediate will be allowed to bind covalently to critical cell constituents and to initiate the pathologic process (Fig. 3–7). The concentration of GSH in rodent lung is about 2 to 4 mM and, apparently, is heterogeneously distributed. Animal experiments indicate a reduction in glutathione S-transferase isoenzyme levels with aging, suggesting that risks of toxic effects from exposure to electrophiles may increase with advancing age.

Although GSH-sensitive alkylation has been well described, additional mechanisms of alkylation also occur, such as nonsensitive GSH electrophilic alkylation and tissue alkylation through radical formation. The site(s) for metabolic formation of reactive intermediates in the respiratory tract would appear to be Clara and alveolar epithelial type II cells, because they are the major sites of cytochrome P_{450}-dependent monooxygenase activity. Several studies have shown that ascorbic acid may be an important component of the lung's defense against metabolically activated toxins. Type II cells and macrophages are the major sites of ascorbic acid uptake.

It is also possible for the lung to undergo injury from a reactive intermediate formed in the liver that reaches the lung through the circulation. Pyrrolizidine alkaloids, for example, are found in various plants hazardous to both animals and humans. Their most prominent toxic effect is liver damage, but the lung is also an important target organ. Highly reactive pyrrole derivatives are believed to be formed in the liver and released into the venous effluent, whereupon they travel to the lung and bind avidly to macromolecular constituents. The result is endothelial injury, with attendant pulmonary edema and pulmonary hypertension.

Tissue alkylation is not the only mechanism of toxicity known to occur in the lung. The herbicide paraquat is a well-known pneumotoxin that can induce lung damage. After being actively taken up by the lung, paraquat is believed to undergo several important modifications. It first undergoes reduction to a free radical by NADPH, a reaction catalyzed by cytochrome c reductase. Secondly, the free radical is reoxidized by oxygen,

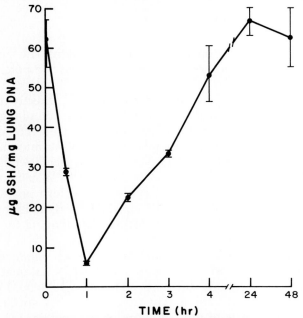

Figure 3–6. Effect of an acute dose (1.0 mg/kg intraperitoneally) of the edematogenic agent thiourea on lung concentration of reduced glutathione (GSH). (From Hollinger, M. A., and Giri, S. N.: ^{14}C-thiourea binding in the rat lung. Res. Commun. Chem. Pathol. Pharmacol. 26:611, 1979.)

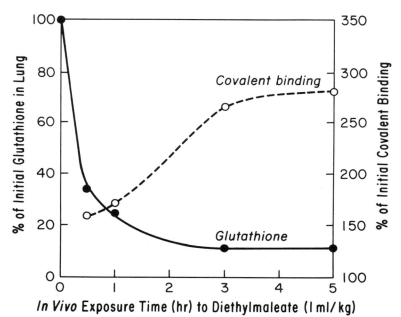

Figure 3–7. Effect of glutathione depletion *in vivo* on covalent binding of radioactivity from ^{14}C-thiourea to lung protein *in vitro*. (From Hollinger, M. A., Giri, S. N., and Hwang, F.: Binding of radioactivity from ^{14}C-thiourea to rat lung protein. Drug Metab. Dispos. 4:121, 1976.)

yielding the paraquat cation and superoxide anion. The generation of superoxide has been hypothesized as having at least two potentially lethal cellular effects.

On the one hand, superoxide anions may lead, directly or indirectly, to lipid peroxidation and to cell death by the production of highly reactive hydroxyl or oxygen radicals. Lipid peroxidation in this context refers to the oxidative destruction of cell membrane polyunsaturated lipids. Alternatively, the continued oxidation of NADPH may deplete this cofactor to the point at which its concentration is too low to sustain other critical cellular functions, such as fatty acid synthesis. A third possibility is that paraquat-induced depletion of NADPH in the lung renders the cells more susceptible to lipid peroxidation by effectively prolonging the life of lipid hydroperoxides (Fig. 3–8).

The involvement of superoxide anion in paraquat toxicity has prompted researchers to try to attenuate the effect of paraquat in the lung by administering superoxide dismutase. This enzyme would presumably inactivate the superoxide anion, but results obtained so far have been conflicting. On the basis of the large size of the protein, it is difficult to understand how it could gain access to the parenchymal cells in which paraquat produces its damage. Interestingly, superoxide dismutase is now displayed in advertisements from health food companies accompanying

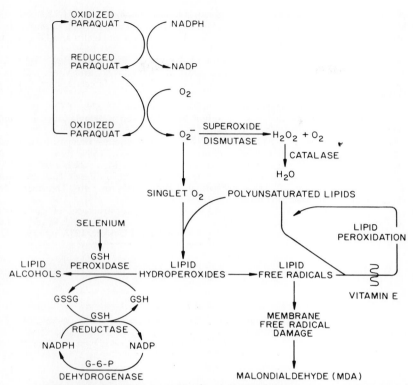

Figure 3–8. Proposed mechanism of paraquat toxicity. (From Bus, J., et al.: A mechanism of paraquat toxicity in mice and rats. Toxicol. Appl. Pharmacol. 35:508, 1976.)

those for vitamins. On the basis of present evidence, there is no justification for self-medication with this product.

Nitrofurantoin-induced lung injury has recently been compared to the injury of lung cells by paraquat. There is biochemical evidence indicating that nitrofurantoin may act like paraquat in evoking an oxidation reduction cycle within lung cells to increase the generation of single electron transfers. The finding that antioxidants can reduce nitrofurantoin-induced lung injury supports the role of oxidant-mediated pathology. Despite similarities, however, it appears that paraquat is much more potent in this regard.

SELECTED REFERENCES

Boyd, M. R.: Metabolic activation of chemical-induced lung disease: implications for the cancer field. *In* Brown, S. S., and Davies, D. S. (eds.): Organ-Directed Toxicity, Chemical Indices and Mechanisms, Oxford, Pergamon Press, pp. 267–272, 1981.

Douglas, J. G., et al.: Pulmonary hypertension and fenfluramine. Br. Med. J., 283:881, 1981.

Ferreira, S. H., and Bakhle, Y. S.: Inactivation of bradykinin and related peptides in the lung. *In* Bakhle, Y. S., and Vane, J. R. (eds.): Lung Biology in Health and Disease, Vol. 4, New York, Marcel Dekker, 1977, pp. 33–53.

Flower, R. J.: Drugs which inhibit prostaglandin biosynthesis. Pharmacol. Rev., 26:33, 1974.

Flower, R. J.: Prostaglandin metabolism in the lung. *In* Bakhle, Y. S., and Vane, J. R. (eds.): Lung Biology in Health and Disease, Vol. 4, New York, Marcel Dekker, 1977, pp. 85–122.

Hook, G. E. R.: Pulmonary metabolism of xenobiotics. Life Sci., 18:279, 1976.

Kuehl, F., Dougherty, H., and Ham, E.: Interactions between prostaglandins and leukotrienes. Biochem. Pharmacol., 33:1, 1984.

Lewis, R. A., and Austen, K. F.: The biologically active leukotrienes: Biosynthesis, metabolism receptors, functions and pharmacology. J. Clin. Invest., 73:889, 1984.

Moncada, S.: Mode of action of aspirin-like drugs. Adv. Intern. Med., 24:1, 1979.

Roth, R.: The lungs and metabolic clearance in health and disease. *In* Benet, L. Z., Massoud, N., and Gambertoglio, J. G. (eds.): Pharmacokinetic Basis for Drug Treatment, New York, Raven Press, 1984, pp. 105–117.

Ryan, V. S., and Ryan, J. W.: Correlations between the five structures of the alveolar-capillary unit and its metabolic activities. *In* Bakhle, Y. S., and Vane, J. R. (eds.): Lung Biology in Health and Disease, Vol. 4, New York, Marcel Dekker, 1977, pp. 197–232.

CHAPTER 4

Antiasthmatic Drugs

ASTHMA

General Considerations

Respiratory pharmacology concerns those drugs that affect the pulmonary system, and the most significant respiratory disorder requiring pharmacologic intervention is undoubtedly asthma. Although numerous definitions of asthma exist, it is clear that asthma, regardless of etiology, is characterized by the following: an increase in airway resistance caused by contraction of bronchiolar smooth muscle, increased bronchiolar secretions, and edema of the bronchiolar mucosa. Asthma is an uncommon cause of death (0.8/100,000 population), but it is a source of severe disability to the approximate 5% of the population that have or have had it.

In the susceptible individual, asthmatic attacks can be elicited by a diverse range of stimuli, including drugs, infection, air pollutants, coughing or laughing, emotional stress, exercise, cold air, and aerosolized distilled water. The situation is complicated because some of the offending agents have widespread exposure as a result of their very nature. For example, it has been estimated that 500,000 or more asthmatics in the United States may be sensitive to sulfites (*e.g.*, sodium or potassium bisulfite or metabisulfite) added to food, drink, and drugs as an antioxidant preservative.

There is disagreement whether antigenic or nonantigenic stimuli account for the majority of all patients experiencing asthmatic symptoms. However, most adults with asthma have no evidence of immediate hypersensitivity to antigens, and most attacks cannot be related to recent exposure to an unusual quantity of antigens. Nevertheless, there are compelling reasons for believing that mediators play a major role in nonallergic forms of asthma as well (the allergic aspect of asthma will be considered in more detail in Chapter 7). The major therapeutic goals of treatment in asthma include correction of bronchospasm, retained secretions, and mucosal edema to decrease the obstruction to air flow.

Etiology

The predominance of airway symptomology is believed to be the result both of hyperresponsiveness of this area to factors that normally produce bronchoconstriction and of an imbalance of autonomic control of bronchiolar tone. The net effect is an exaggeration of the parasympathetic response and a reduction in the effectiveness of the sympathetic broncho-dilator mechanism. It is a common clinical observation that β agonists also become less effective as asthmatic episodes become more severe.

Specifically, it has been suggested that asthmatics may have an acquired or inherited defect in their lung β_2 receptors. This attractive hypothesis is supported by the observation that asthmatics are particularly sensitive to β_2-blocking drugs. In such patients, intense bronchoconstric-tion can occur with normal doses of the blocker, suggesting an inordinate degree of receptor occupancy. Here again, the effect would be to reduce an already diminished ability to antagonize parasympathetic control.

It is also possible that sensory receptors in the airways of asthmatic patients are themselves hypersensitive to endogenous chemical mediators. In this regard, sensitivity to acetylcholine and histamine is elevated tenfold in the asthmatic, whereas the sensitivity to PGF_2 is reported to be approximately 10,000-fold greater.

The principal drugs currently used in the treatment of asthma are of four pharmacologic types: the sympathomimetic bronchodilators; the-ophylline and its derivatives; the anti-inflammatory steroids; and sodium cromoglycate. The choice of type of agent and route of administration depends on individual patient need and tolerance.

SYMPATHOMIMETIC BRONCHODILATORS

The sympathomimetic group of bronchodilators has been effectively used for the treatment of asthma since the end of the 19th century, and they are probably still the most widely used antiasthmatic drugs. They are particularly effective against mild and occasional episodic asthma—that is, mild symptoms (wheezing and dyspnea) occurring less than 2 or 3 days each month. Drugs in this group combine with two basic types of sympathetic system receptors, α and β, and the β receptors can be further subdivided into β_1 and β_2 subtypes. Characteristic effects produced by the interaction of sympathomimetic drugs and these receptors, with particular emphasis on selected sites pertinent to the respiratory system, are shown in Table 4-1.

On the basis of these effects, it would appear desirable to use a sympathomimetic drug with preferential affinity for β_2 receptors (bron-chodilation and inhibition of histaminic release) and minimal affinity for α (bronchoconstriction) and β_1 (cardiovascular) receptors. The develop-ment of β_2-stimulant bronchodilators was a consequence of the recognition

Table 4–1. Selected α- and β-Receptor Effects

Site	α	β₁	β₂
Arterioles	Vasoconstriction		Vasodilation
Tracheobronchial smooth muscle	Possible bronchoconstriction		Bronchodilation
Heart	Reflex bradycardia	Tachycardia plus inotropism	
Mast cells	Enhanced histamine release		Inhibition of histamine release
Other			Skeletal muscle tremors

of the limitations of epinephrine and isoproterenol as bronchodilators. Table 4-2 lists the major sympathomimetic drugs used as bronchodilators and compares their relative receptor affinities. The availability of these new analogs have made epinephrine, ephedrine, and isoproterenol, with their normal receptor affinities, increasingly redundant in the routine management of asthma. However, because these agents have been historically the "classic" sympathomimetic drugs used in asthma, all newer drugs are usually compared to them.

Drugs

Epinephrine is the standard against which most sympathomimetics are judged. It is a powerful bronchodilator, whether given by injection or inhalation. Unfortunately, it stimulates both α and β receptors. Therefore,

Table 4–2. Comparison of Receptor Preference for Major Sympathomimetic Bronchodilator Drugs*

Drug	Main Route(s) of Administration	Receptor Site Preference		
		α	β₁	β₂
Ephedrine	Oral Subcutaneous Intramuscular Intravenous	2+	3+	3+
Epinephrine	Subcutaneous	3+	4+	3+
	Intramuscular	3+	4+	3+
	Inhalation	3+	4+	3+
Isoproterenol	Inhalation		4+	4+
Isoetharine	Inhalation		1+	3+
Metaproterenol	Inhalation		1+	3+
	Oral		1+	3+
Terbutaline	Subcutaneous		1+	3+
	Oral		1+	3+
Albuterol	Inhalation		1+	4+
	Oral		1+	4+

*These are relative approximations, in which 1+ indicates a minor effect while 4 + indicates a strong effect.

its effects on the cardiovascular system can be dangerous, and may outweigh its benefits. This is particularly true in the elderly and in others with known cardiovascular disease. Repeated use has also been reported to lead to tolerance. Currently, the major indication for the use of epinephrine in treating bronchospasm is in the therapy of acute anaphylaxis. Epinephrine is administered primarily by injection (usually subcutaneously) for this use. The use of epinephrine aerosol has been declining recently with the introduction of more specific bronchiolar smooth muscle agonists.

Ephedrine was one of the first drugs to be used for bronchodilation, and is still present in many preparations. Its major disadvantages are also related to its mixed α- and β-agonist activity. This manifests itself with undesirable cardiovascular and central nervous system effects. Ephedrine also has a tendency to produce mucosal drying and urinary retention, which is of particular concern to elderly men with benign prostate hypertrophy. An advantage of ephedrine has been its oral effectiveness. Unfortunately, it has a relatively short duration of action but, when given with theophylline, the duration of action of ephedrine has been reported to be comparable to that of terbutaline (see below) or of higher doses of theophylline. The current use of ephedrine appears to be declining with the advent of orally acting selective β_2 agonists.

Isoproterenol is a mixed β_1 and β_2 agonist with negligible α effects. Although specific for β receptors, its role as a bronchodilator is limited by its affinity for β_1 receptors. When used, isoproterenol is best administered in the form of an aerosol so that it is concentrated at the site of action, and the possibility of systemic cardiovascular effects is minimized. It has a rapid onset of action, about 2 to 5 minutes, with a short duration of action (1 to 1½ hours) because of its rapid inactivation. The use of isoproterenol aerosols has also declined recently since the introduction of the selective β_2 bronchodilators.

As mentioned above, several new drugs have been introduced during the last few years that have two main advantages as bronchodilators: prolonged activity and increased β_2 selectivity. These characteristics were produced by modification of the benzene ring (movement of the hydroxyl from position 4 to 5 or substitution for the hydroxyl at position 3) and substitution on the amine head, respectively. A comparison of the chemical structures of important bronchodilator sympathomimetic amines is shown in Figure 4-1.

Isoetharine is a commonly used fast-acting bronchodilator about 10% as potent as isoproterenol on human bronchial smooth muscle. However, because its cardiovascular effects are only 1/300 as potent as those of isoproterenol, its β_2:β_1 ratio is approximately 30 times greater. Isoetharine is only available in the aerosol form in the United States.

Metaproterenol is a derivative of isoproterenol that is resistant to catechol-o-methyltransferase (COMT) and has, therefore, a longer duration of action than isoproterenol. It is approximately as effective as isoproterenol when administered by inhalation. When given orally, it is at least as effective as terbutaline and albuterol, although possibly more prone to increase heart rate.

Terbutaline and albuterol (salbutamol) are so similar in their pharmacology and therapeutic applications that they are often discussed together. Like metaproterenol, these drugs are not subject to inactivation by COMT, which explains their longer duration of action (3 to 7 hours, depending on route of administration). These and other β_2 agents would appear to possess potential therapeutic advantages over less selective β-receptor bronchodilators. Because of their β_2 agonism, these drugs also inhibit histamine release from mast cells, produce vasodilation, and increase ciliary motility.

β-Receptor selectivity by other drugs can also be important to the asthmatic. For example, propranolol has been widely used in the management of angina pectoris and cardiac arrhythmias because of its blocking effect on β_1 receptors. Unfortunately, propranolol also has some β_2-receptor blocking activity, which often aggravates bronchospasm in asthmatics receiving the drug. A more specific β_1 blocker such as metoprolol would seem to be a better choice in the management of asthmatics suffering from angina pectoris and cardiac arrhythmias. Sympathomimetic bronchodilators may be less effective in elderly patients because of reduced β-receptor affinity. However, tolerance to β_2-bronchodilator action is not a routine problem in the management of asthmatics.

Aerosol Administration

The use of bronchodilator aerosols, whether by metered-dose inhaler or by nebulized solution, is a popular route of administration for these

Chemical Structures of Important Bronchodilator Sympathomimetic Amines

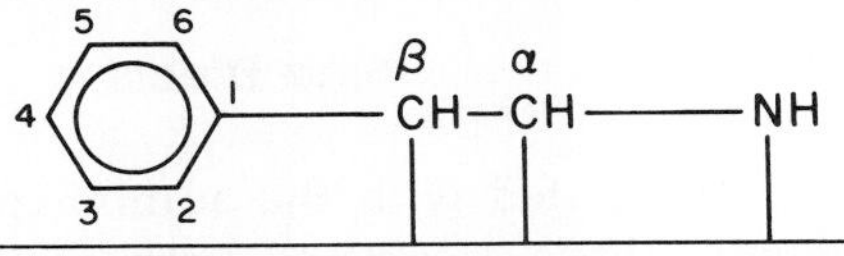

		β	α	
Epinephrine	3-OH, 4-OH	OH	H	CH_3
Isoproterenol	3-OH, 4-OH	OH	H	$CH(CH_3)_2$
Isoetharine	3-OH, 4-OH	OH	CH_2CH_3	$CH(CH_3)_2$
Metaproterenol	3-OH, 5-OH	OH	H	$CH(CH_3)_2$
Terbutaline	3-OH, 5-OH	OH	H	$C(CH_3)_3$
Salbutamol	3-CH_2OH, 4-OH	OH	H	$C(CH_3)_3$
Ephedrine		OH	CH_3	CH_3

Figure 4–1. Structural relationship of phenylethylamine substitutions to α and β receptor agonism.

agents that is associated with certain advantages and disadvantages. Advantages include the need for a lower dose (5 to 10%), more reliable absorption than use of the gastric route, and a more rapid response rate. Disadvantages include the following: the need to generate drug-carrying particles in the range of 1 to 5 μm in diameter to reach the small bronchi (90% of the "inhaled" dose is routinely swallowed); variations in technique, such as rate of inhalation and duration of breath holding, can influence the amount of drug deposited; ineffective administration via aerosol in pre-existing bronchospasm (smaller surface area with excess secretion); possibility of overadministration as a result of failure to follow instructions (particularly in children and the elderly); abuse potential, with difficulty in substituting alternative bronchodilator treatment; and potential cardiac hazard if the propellant (halogenated hydrocarbons) is used injudiciously. The following is a summary of the most effective way to use a metered dose inhaler:

1. Shake the cannister thoroughly.
2. Place the mouthpiece of the actuator between the lips.
3. Breathe out steadily.
4. Fire the inhaler while taking a slow deep inhalation.
5. Hold the breath at full inspiration for 10 seconds.

There is also continued interest in combining aerosol administration with other routes of administration to achieve greater bronchodilation. For example, because aerosols are normally deposited in the most dilated airways, they will not be delivered where they are needed most. Delivery to the lungs by drugs given orally or parenterally is dependent on the vascular status, though, so combining these routes could conceivably achieve a higher degree of airway access. Unfortunately, no well-controlled studies have been carried out. Nonetheless, it appears that β_2 stimulants given by inhalation combine maximal effectiveness with minimal side effect liability, and these should be considered as the drugs of choice.

Side Effects

Side effects associated with the administration of sympathomimetic agents are usually those associated with α and β_1 effects, and include nervousness, headache, tachycardia, palpitations, nausea, vomiting, and sweating. In general, these relatively mild symptoms appear to decrease with chronic therapy.

β_2-Selective bronchodilators are without significant side effects when taken by inhalation at the recommended dose. If taken by mouth, both skeletal muscle tremor and tachycardia may be seen. To date it has not been possible to produce an efficacious, selective β_2-sympathomimetic bronchodilator that is devoid of this action when administered systemically. Fortunately, these tremors decrease with prolonged use of the drug. The origin of the tachycardia is probably a reflex in response to peripheral vasodilation, although some minimal direct effect on the heart is possible. In any event, cardiovascular responses to albuterol, for example, are generally innocuous to the extent that suicide attempts with this drug have been characteristically unsuccessful.

Hypoxemia has also been described as an ironic complication of sympathomimetic therapy in some patients. The decrease in oxygenation of the blood appears to result from a drug-induced general increase in pulmonary blood flow (vasodilation) to all areas of the lungs. Because this can include shunting of the blood to areas that are poorly ventilated, a net decrease in the ventilation-to-perfusion ratio can occur. Generally, an adrenergic aerosol-induced fall in the arterial pressure of oxygen (PaO_2) is not clinically significant. However, in some cases, if blood oxygen is already low (e.g., $PaO_2 < 60$ mm Hg), oxygen may be administered with the bronchodilator. Parenteral use of albuterol or terbutaline in pregnant women for the treatment of asthma may delay the onset of labor.

Mechanism of Action

The beneficial effects of sympathomimetic drugs in the treatment of asthma appear to be primarily related to the elevation of cyclic AMP (cAMP) levels in bronchial smooth muscle, as described in Chapter 1. This is a consequence of their activation of adenylate cyclase, which is part of the β_2 receptor (Fig. 4-2). The result is an increase in the cAMP concentration and subsequent activation of cAMP-dependent protein-

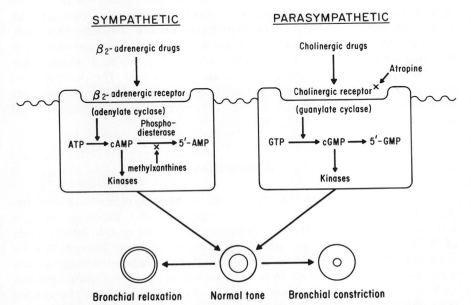

Figure 4-2. Comparison of sympathetic and parasympathetic receptor activation on bronchial smooth muscle tone.

kinase, which leads, in an unknown way, to relaxation of bronchial smooth muscle. An additional advantageous effect of β_2 agonists is prevention of mast cell disruption with the release of endogenous bronchoconstrictor substances. As noted above, asthmatics are hyperresponsive to many antigenic factors. An additional advantage of β_2 agonists is that they can increase tracheal mucociliary transport, and in this way possibly hasten the elimination of bronchial secretions.

METHYLXANTHINE BRONCHODILATORS

In addition to sympathomimetic drugs, methylxanthines such as theophylline (1,3-dimethylxanthine) have played an important role in the acute and chronic management of the asthmatic patient. Theophylline has been used as a primary or first-line drug in the treatment of chronic asthma in the United States. It has found particular favor in cases of moderate to severe asthma, in which maintenance therapy is essential (*i.e.*, distressing episodes with a frequency of more than two per week).

Although introduced approximately 50 years ago, it is only recently that the popularity of theophylline has begun to grow. Sales figures from 1977 indicated that 42% of all prescriptions written for bronchodilators were for theophylline products. The market for bronchial therapy in the United States was estimated to be over $300 million in 1983.

Effects of theophylline on the airway are similar to those produced by β_2 agonists, and include smooth muscle relaxation, inhibition of mast cell degranulation, and an increase in mucociliary transport rate. Theophylline itself has a powerful relaxant effect on bronchial smooth muscle, and a number of different types of preparations are available. However, because the theophylline molecule itself is nonpolar, it has very poor aqueous solubility. Therefore, more soluble derivatives such as the ethylenediamine salt (aminophylline) are usually employed. The development of improved pharmaceutic preparations and the availability of methods for measuring blood (and salivary) levels have contributed to the renewed interest in the use of theophylline.

Clinical Uses

The various commercial theophylline analogs differ in their theophylline content and pharmaceutic composition and, therefore, in their pharmacokinetics and pharmacodynamics. Sustained-release formulations of theophylline can prolong the effective life of a dose of theophylline by extending its absorption from the intestinal tract. This technology avoids the many peaks and valleys in serum levels that are seen during frequent dosing with immediate-release products, and also lengthens the dosing interval.

Some preparations containing aminophylline have been given an enteric coating because aminophylline can cause severe gastric irritation when taken orally. When taken by mouth, theophylline preparations have a more variable action than sympathomimetic bronchodilators because of their solubility problem. The pharmaceutic ingenuity that has been invested in these various theophylline preparations originated primarily in the United States. This situation reflects the dependence of American physicians on theophylline, because the β_2-stimulant bronchodilators available in Europe for years have only recently become available in the United States.

All theophylline capsules or tablets require multiple daily doses over a 24-hour period, which undoubtedly contributes to variability in blood plasma levels because of patient noncompliance. The FDA has approved the first once-daily oral theophylline (Theo-24), and this new prescription product will be available in a controlled-release capsule dosage form (100-300 mg). It is claimed that this product will maintain therapeutic blood plasma levels of theophylline for a full 24 hours.

Aminophylline is highly effective, with a rapid onset of action when given intravenously. Therefore, intravenous aminophylline is especially valuable as the first-line treatment in cases of status asthmaticus. The consensus of clinical pharmacologists is that the therapeutic serum level of theophylline is in the range of 10 to 20 µg/ml. In status asthmaticus, this can be achieved with an initial loading dose of about 5 mg/kg body weight administered intravenously over 30 minutes. This is, of course, calculated on the basis of theophylline content of the preparation being used, which can vary (Table 4-3). The loading dose is followed by a continuous infusion at a rate of approximately 0.6 mg/kg/hour.

Theophylline can also be administered chronically for the maintenance of airway patency in selected patients, and it is usually given orally in such situations. Fortunately, most patients respond well to standard tablet preparations. Patients maintained on prolonged oral doses of theophylline usually show reduced chronic obstruction. As with the acute use of theophylline, the goal of chronic therapy is to achieve a satisfactory blood level.

Individuals can vary greatly in their serum theophylline levels follow-

Table 4-3. Comparison of Theophylline Content of Various Preparations

Preparation	% Theophylline	Equivalent Dosage (mg)
Theophylline anhydrous	100	100
Theophylline monohydrate	91	110
Aminophylline anhydrous	86	116
Aminophylline dihydrate	79	127
Oxtriphylline	64	156
Theophylline sodium glycinate	49	200
Theophylline calcium salicylate	48	208

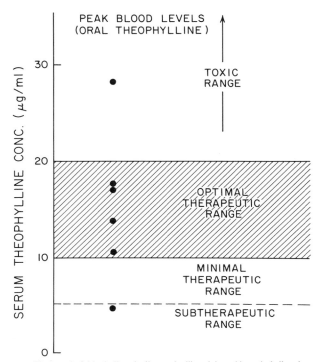

Figure 4–3. Variation in theophylline blood levels following oral administration of an equal oral dose (mg/kg) to six individuals.

ing administration of a standard oral dose of the drug, and even among healthy subjects in controlled environments there is wide variation in metabolism. Various medical conditions and environmental variables have been shown to influence its uptake. Figure 4-3 shows blood levels that the clinician might expect when an equal milligram-to-kilogram oral dose is given to various subjects, and illustrates the narrow optimal serum range. In principle, any theophylline or aminophylline preparation can be used in maintenance therapy, because there is no compelling evidence for choosing one preparation over another, except for comparative cost (aminophylline preparations are less expensive). The new once-daily preparation may prove an exception to this generalization.

Alternatives to oral tablets include elixirs, nonalcoholic solutions, and rectal suppositories; the latter can be used for prolonged absorption, especially overnight. However, absorption is variable, and proctitis occasionally occurs. These preparations are generally used when tablets are unacceptable or in emergency situations. A comparison of different types of theophylline and aminophylline preparations is given in Table 4-4.

There are also a number of combination preparations on the market containing theophylline or a derivative, and one or more additional agents.

Ephedrine and phenobarbital are the most popular ingredients, although antacids and expectorants may also be present. In each case, a rational argument for their inclusion can undoubtedly be made by the manufacturer. However, the most intelligent approach, based on sound pharmacologic principles, is generally to avoid fixed-dose combination products.

It should be remembered when determining theophylline dosage that various factors can either increase or decrease the required dosage. For example, heavy cigarette smoking may require a 50 to 100% increase in dosage; this is probably the result of cytochrome P_{450} enzyme induction by inhalation of polycyclic hydrocarbons. On the other hand, pre-existing congestive heart failure and severe liver disease decrease the elimination of theophylline and, therefore, lower doses should be used to avoid accumulation of toxic levels (see Table 4-5 for additional details). This is a particular problem in the elderly. Similarly, drugs such as cimetidine and erythromycin can inhibit theophylline metabolism, leading to increased

Table 4–4. Theophylline and Aminophylline Preparations

Preparation	General Comments
Theophylline	
Tablet and capsules	Tablets should be regarded as a drug of first choice; a new long-acting preparation (24 hours) is available that offers the advantage of once-daily dosage: microencapsulated and sustained-release beads have been found to be useful in treating children
Solutions	Elixirs containing theophylline dissolved in 20% ethanol are available; although effective and rapid absorption can occur, elixirs probably do not provide any advantages over other liquid or solid preparations; products containing less alcohol are appropriate for children, who should not receive elixirs.
Suppositories	These have rapid and erratic absorption; they are usually used in emergency situations; the monoethanolamine derivative is more soluble and is used in the enema preparations.
Inhalation	The saturated aqueous solution is well tolerated but is not very effective as compared to sympathomimetics.
Aminophylline	
Intravenous	Aminophylline is used mainly as an intravenous drug for the management of acute bronchospasm; it should not be administered rapidly but over 10 to 15 minutes.
Tablets and capsules	Tablets can be used successfuly for chronic therapy, and equivalent doses are less expensive than theophylline; enteric-coated preparations do not appear to be well absorbed, and their use is discouraged.
Rectal suppositories and solutions	Suppositories are generally not preferred because of erratic absorption, low blood levels, and irritation; there are some patients, however, who do respond favorably, with a minimum of gastric side effects; enema preparations are available that can be used twice daily for many years, either prophylactically or therapeutically; patients who are prone to asthma attacks can use this route instead of the intravenous.
Inhalation	Aminophylline powder has been reported to be of some value, but its use has been abandoned; an aqueous solution is irritating and of little proven value.

Table 4–5. Factors Altering Theophylline Dosage*

Situations Requiring Increased Dosage	Situations Requiring Decreased Dosage
Children 2 months to 16 years old	Premature neonates (theophylline treatment rarely justified)
Cigarette smokers and patients exposed to hydrocarbon fumes	Elderly patients with borderline cardiac and hepatic function
Patients with suboptimal blood levels, or blood levels below 10 µg/ml	Cirrhosis, hepatic insufficiency
Patients with acidosis (possibly)	Heart failure, cor pulmonale, acute pulmonary edema
Patients known to have a high tolerance to theophylline, (*i.e.*, rapid metabolizers)	Patients who manifest toxic symptoms on standard dosage
Patients on high-protein diets	Patients who have received theophylline therapy in previous 24 hours
	Patients with alkalosis (possibly)
	Patients with fever and toxemia
	Patients taking a macrolide antibiotic (*e.g.*, troleandomycin and erythromycins) or an H_2 antagonist (*e.g.*, cimetidine and ranitidine)

*(Modified from Ziment, I.: Respiratory Pharmacology and Therapeutics, Philadelphia, W. B. Saunders, 1978, p. 194.)

blood levels and risk of toxicity. In effect, because the half-life of theophylline varies among patients, appropriate dosage schedules should ideally be developed for each patient. It was the variation in patient response that contributed to the erratic results obtained with early theophylline preparations.

Side Effects

Achieving the correct dosage in a given patient is extremely important, because theophylline therapy has a relatively narrow therapeutic range. Young or old patients and those with abnormal theophylline metabolism require the most careful dosing. Serum theophylline levels of inpatients should be checked either on an alternate-day basis, or when drug dosages are changed. Outpatient levels should be checked when the clinical response is not optimal, clinical toxicity is suspected, or a drug such as cimetidine is started or stopped. Saliva rather than serum has reportedly been used for determining theophylline levels: saliva theophylline levels are approximately 50% of those of serum.

Treatment with theophylline preparations is associated with certain undesirable side effects (Table 4-6). The appearance and character of these reactions is related to the serum level of theophylline. At serum concentrations lower than 20 µg/ml, 85% of patients are free of serious toxic effects. The most frequent side effects encountered are anorexia, nausea, vomiting and abdominal discomfort, headache, anxiety, and nervousness. Serious cardiac, CNS, or respiratory toxicity is associated with rapid intravenous injection leading to high levels in brain or heart and with plasma theophylline concentrations higher than 30 μg/ml. Monitoring of plasma concentration is, therefore, of great importance during intravenous administration.

Mechanism of Action

The bronchodilator effect of theophylline and its derivatives is usually ascribed to its ability to inhibit cyclic nucleotide phosphodiesterase, which normally hydrolyzes cAMP. In this way, intracellular levels of cAMP would be expected to rise and, in effect, would achieve the same result as the sympathomimetics (see Fig. 4-2). Although this is an attractive hypothesis, more definitive experiments must be carried out to explain certain inconsistencies. For example, maximal therapeutic concentrations of theophylline have been found to inhibit tissue phosphodiesterase activity by only about 5% *in vitro*.

Theophylline is known to stimulate the release of catecholamines from the adrenal medulla, as well as to inhibit catechol-O-methyltransferase and histamine release from mast cells. Additional evidence suggests that theophylline can antagonize the bronchoconstriction effect of PGF_2 or act on the cell membrane. Another beneficial effect of theophylline is to increase mucociliary clearance. Perhaps these effects or a direct action contribute to its bronchodilator action.

Because phosphodiesterase inhibitors and β_2-sympathomimetic drugs are thought to produce bronchodilation by increasing intracellular cAMP levels, there has been interest in combined treatment with these agents.

Table 4–6. Major Adverse Effects of Theophylline Therapy

Adverse Effect	Serum Level	Comments
Anorexia, nausea, vomiting	About 15 μg/ml or higher	Most common; more likely with oral preparations, suggesting effect on gastric mucosa; incidence varies with preparation
Cardiovascular	>30 μg/ml	Mainly with intravenous aminophylline; too rapid injection can lead to cardiac arrest, palpitations, tachycardia, and arrhythmias; also, hypertension or hypotension may occur
Central nervous system	>40 μg/ml	Drug-induced seizures with intravenous aminophylline, especially in children; respiratory arrest has been reported
Allergy	Not dose-related	Usually rashes, although anaphylaxis can occur; probably caused by ethylenediamine component

Most clinical studies carried out to date in asthmatic patients indicate that treatment with oral or intravenous theophylline and with oral or inhaled β_2 agents has an additive effect. These results lead to two conclusions, therefore: the combination of both should produce bronchodilation at lower respective doses than either drug alone; and theophylline is not acting as a phosphodiesterase inhibitor, because a synergistic effect would be expected if this were the case.

Recent studies also indicate that the respiratory stimulant effect of methylxanthines may involve interaction with adenosine receptors in the central nervous system. Under normal circumstances, adenosine functions as a neuromodulator to decrease respiration by binding primarily to an A_2 subset of receptors. It has been hypothesized that the central respiratory stimulant effect of methylxanthines (*e.g.*, theophylline) is a product of their antagonism of adenosine for these receptors. In addition, it is also believed that theophylline acts as a bronchodilator by antagonizing the inhibitory effect of adenosine on adenylate cyclase in airway smooth muscle cells. The result of this effect would be an increase in intracellular cAMP levels and smooth muscle relaxation.

Caffeine

Caffeine (1,3,7-trimethylxanthine) is closely related in chemical structure and pharmacologic activity to theophylline. A double-blind clinical study indicates that a single oral dose of caffeine (10 mg/kg) can be as effective a bronchodilator as theophylline (5 mg/kg) in young patients with asthma. Although not recommended for regular use as a bronchodilator, caffeine may have value for temporary use as a bronchodilator when prescribed antiasthmatic medications are not readily available. A patient weighing 70 kg would have to drink five to seven cups of average coffee (containing 100 to 150 mg caffeine per cup) to obtain a bronchodilator effect.

GLUCOCORTICOIDS

The adrenal cortex produces a group of steroids known as glucocorticoids, the most notable of which is cortisol. The principal physiologic functions of cortisol involve carbohydrate, protein, and lipid regulation. During the 1930s, the observation was made that pregnant women with arthritis experienced symptomatic relief of joint pain during their pregnancy. It was believed that adrenocortical secretions were responsible, and this led to the discovery of the anti-inflammatory effect of glucocorticoids. Subsequently, derivatives of cortisol were developed that preserved the anti-inflammatory effect while minimizing electrolyte-related side effects. Glucocorticoids have been used to treat asthma since 1950.

Mechanism of Action

The palliative effect of glucocorticoids in bronchial asthma is probably related to their anti-inflammatory properties. Glucocorticoids can interfere with the inflammatory process at several points (Table 4-7). However, the precise mechanism(s) by which glucocorticoids reverse airway constriction is unknown. The most logical explanation may involve steroid alteration of catecholamines and their receptors, resulting in enhanced sympathomimetic responsiveness of airway smooth muscle.

Recently, an important observation was made that may provide the best explanation for the mechanism of action of glucocorticoids. It is now known that glucocorticoids induce the formation of a protein referred to as lipomodulin, whose function is the inhibition of phospholipase A_2 action on membrane phospholipids. The result is a decrease in the availability of arachidonic acid for prostaglandin and leukotriene formation (see Chap. 3). Thus, potent smooth muscle spasmogens are prevented from being synthesized.

Clinical Uses

The appropriate role of glucocorticoids in the therapy of asthma has become somewhat clearer in recent years. Today, glucocorticoid use is generally reserved for the asthmatic with troublesome symptoms despite full therapy. The safest use of these agents is for the acute treatment of

Table 4-7. General Anti-Inflammatory Effects of Glucocorticoids*

Action	Significance
Maintains microcirculation (vasoconstriction) by suppression of kinin activity	Prevents leakage of fluid from blood vessels, with formation of tissue edema
Inhibits migration of leukocytes and mast cells	Decreases exudation and migration of inflammatory cells (e.g., phagocytes, macrophages)
Reduces polymorph stickiness and margination in blood vessels	Impairs polymorph activity
Causes lymphopenia, monocytopenia, eosinopenia	Unknown
Maintains cell membrane integrity	Protects cells from damage by noxious events; prevents intracellular sequestration of water that would swell and damage cells
Stabilizes lysosomal membranes in such structures as mast cells	Prevents release of mediators that induce inflammatory reactions
Reduces tissue stores of histamine and other mediators	Decreases availability of mediators that cause inflammatory reaction
Potentiates catecholamine activity	Enhances sympathomimetic responsiveness
Enhances cardiac inotropy and improves circulatory function	Improves cardiopulmonary function in conditions of severe stress, such as shock

*(From Ziment, I.: Respiratory Pharmacology and Therapeutics, Philadelphia, W. B. Saunders, 1978, p. 221.)

the severely ill patient with status asthmaticus. These hormones should not be employed in any asthmatic condition that can be brought under moderate control with other measures. In particular, chronic steroid use should be minimized and avoided whenever possible; this is particularly true with children.

The reason for this warning is the potential of glucocorticoids to produce significant side effects when administered chronically at pharmacologic doses—that is, in excess of the normal 25- to 40-mg daily cortisol output. These complications involve numerous systems, and can range from merely unpleasant to dangerous (Table 4-8). Glucocorticoid use is

Table 4–8. Complications That May Be Associated with Glucocorticoid Therapy*

Site or System Affected	Unpleasant Effects	Dangerous Effects
Skin	Acne, hirsutism, striae, flushing, facial erythema, increased perspiration	Loss of subcutaneous tissue, poor wound healing
Vascular	Petechiae, bruising	Thromboemboli, vasculitis, periarteritis nodosa
Appearance	Fat deposition (facial mooning, buffalo hump)	Stunting of growth in children
Central nervous system	Insomnia, restlessness, agitation, nocturia	Altered personality, psychosis (euphoria, mania, depression, confusion), pseudotumor cerebri
Cardiovascular	Edema (caused by sodium retention)	Hypertension, heart failure, arrhythmias
Metabolic	Electrolyte disturbance, calcium loss, alkalosis, negative nitrogen balance, hyperlipidemia	Diabetogenic effect, hyperosmolar nonketotic coma
Musculoskeletal	Weakness (caused by myopathy, hypokalemia, wasting), osteoporosis	Vertebral and other fractures, aseptic bone necrosis of femoral and humeral heads
Endocrine	Menstrual disorders, menopausal symptoms, impotence	Hypothalamic-pituitary-adrenal axis suppression
Gastrointestinal	Nausea, vomiting, fatty liver, increased appetite, esophagitis	Increased risk of peptic ulceration (in rheumatoid arthritis), large bowel perforation, pancreatitis
Ocular	Exophthalmos, posterior subcapsular cataract, sixth nerve palsies (diplopia)	Papilledema, increased risk of fungal and viral keratitis
Immunologic	Suppression of skin responses to antigenic tests, depression of immunologic responses	Impaired response to infection, susceptibility to dissemination of vaccinations, opportunistic infections
Fetus		Risk of teratogenicity in first trimester, possible adrenal insufficiency in neonate

*(From Ziment, I.: Respiratory Pharmacology and Therapeutics, Philadelphia, W. B. Saunders, 1978, p. 226.)

contraindicated in children and in patients with uncontrolled peptic ulcer, osteoporosis, or psychosis, as well as severe diabetes mellitus, susceptibility to infection, glaucoma, and cataract, unless there is no viable alternative.

There are a number of glucocorticoids available for use in the treatment of asthma (Table 4-9). Because asthmatic attacks vary in their frequency, onset, intensity, and duration, treatment modes vary. In general, a few select preparations are sufficient for treatment of most cases of asthma. In status asthmaticus, for example, if use of a glucocorticoid is desired, a reasonable regimen involves the administration of cortisol (hydrocortisone sodium succinate injection USP) in a loading dose of 4 mg/kg/hour given intravenously over a period of 8 to 10 hours. Adequate plasma levels can then be maintained if an infusion is delivered at the rate of 1 mg/kg/hour. In addition, this method of continuous infusion is less likely to produce electrolyte disturbances (*e.g.*, calcium or

Table 4–9. Glucocorticoids Used in the Treatment of Asthma*

Drug	Advantages	Disadvantages
Cortisol (sodium succinate salt)	Standard intravenous therapy effective in status asthmaticus	May cause electrolyte disturbance
Prednisolone	Fairly rapid acting when given by mouth	Slightly more expensive than prednisone
Prednisone	Standard oral preparation; inexpensive, effective	Not as effective in patients with liver disease
Methylprednisolone	Rapid acting; minimal mineralocorticoid side effects; unproven advantages in severe disease	Relatively expensive
Triamcinolone	Potent; minimal mineralocorticoid side effects; not likely to produce weight gain (acetonide used as aerosol; see below)	May cause myopathy and mental depression
Dexamethasone	Potent; minimal mineralocorticoid side effects; suitable for topical therapy	May markedly stimulate appetite; value in asthma has been controversial
Beclomethasone†	Potent; minimal mineralocorticoid side effects; diproprionate used as aerosol; not very active by oral route	Aerosol may cause hoarseness and oral candidiasis
Betamethasone†	Similar to, but more potent than, dexamethasone; valerate used as aerosol; less potent than beclomethasone dipropionate	Aerosol may cause hoarseness and oral candidiasis; may cause greater adrenal suppression than beclomethasone
Triamcinolone† acetonide	Delivers higher percentage of dose to the airways; may have lower incidence of oral candidiasis	Aerosol may cause hoarseness, wheezing, cough

*(Modified from Ziment, I.: Respiratory Pharmacology and Therapeutics, Philadelphia, W. B. Saunders, 1978, p. 243.)

†Suitable for inhalational administration in asthma, but should not be employed for the treatment of cases of severe status asthmaticus in which intensive measures are required.

potassium loss), and allows plasma cortisol concentrations to be sustained with a smaller total daily dosage than with intermittent injections.

The response to cortisol will probably not be immediate, and may require several hours before becoming apparent. During this interval, it would be appropriate to give a rapidly acting sympathomimetic by inhalation, as well as intravenous aminophylline, if needed. In most cases, control of a severe asthma attack can be achieved within 1 to 3 days. Serious side effects are unlikely to occur during this period, even if heroic doses of the steroid are used. This includes feedback inhibition of the pituitary, allowing rapid tapering, or even abrupt withdrawal of the steroid.

Mild asthma with intermittent symptoms is not treated with gluco-corticoids because the benefits do not justify the risk. Inhaled β_2 agonists are usually sufficient to provide adequate treatment, with minor incon-venience and few side effects. Oral therapy, if necessary, can include agents such as terbutaline or albuterol, or they may be used in combination with theophylline in series or coincidently. A variation on the combination theme popular with some clinicians is the use of a β_2 agonist (*e.g.*, albuterol) aerosol together with oral theophylline. The use of glucocorti-coids should be considered only when the above measures have failed, and when chronic use is unavoidable.

Prednisone and prednisolone are the preferred oral glucocorticoids. The two most relevant considerations in deciding which to use are cost (prednisolone is somewhat more expensive) and metabolism (prednisone is metabolized by the liver to prednisolone). Both drugs are available in a range of concentrations, including enteric-coated preparations.

A recent report indicates that glucocorticoids vary in their ability to penetrate lung tissue. In that study, human volunteers with various lung diseases (including asthma) were treated with steroids orally and then underwent bronchoalveolar lavage. Analysis of the lavage fluid indicated that methylprednisolone passes across the endothelium into lung tissue to a greater extent, and with less variability, than prednisone. This fact has been suggested as a possible explanation for the superior response of patients with idiopathic pulmonary fibrosis to methylprednisolone than to prednisone. Whether this fact is significant in the relief of asthmatic symptoms is not clear, because presumably acute attacks involve smooth muscle higher in the respiratory system rather than parenchymal tissue.

Side Effects

The major difficulties produced by chronic glucocorticoid administra-tion are the result of chronic administration of pharmacologic doses for approximately 2 weeks or more. The greater the increment by which exogenous glucocorticoid exceeds daily cortisol output, the more likely is the incidence of toxicity. All or some of the side effects described previously can occur, depending on the situation. One of the most significant side effects unique to glucocorticoid hormones is hypothalamic-pituitary-adrenal axis feedback disturbance, which can result in acute adrenal insufficiency and resulting sequelae if withdrawal is too rapid. A number of strategies have been devised to minimize the occurrence of this possibility, including various tapering schedules as well as alternate-day steroid therapy.

Attempts have also been made to reduce the side effects of glucocorticoids by using aerosol preparations. Both betamethasone valerate and beclomethasone dipropionate have been found to be effective in relieving asthmatic symptoms without producing significant evidence of adrenal suppression. The latter drug is about twice as potent, and seems to be the preferred preparation.

Both drugs are delivered by metered dose from pressurized containers holding about 200 "puffs." Because the usual regimen for both drugs is two puffs four times a day, an aerosol should last 25 days. Up to 30 puffs of beclomethasone daily (1.5 mg) have been administered without systemic toxicity. However, at higher doses, these agents have also been found to be capable of suppressing local immune mechanisms in the oropharynx, leading to growth of *Candida albicans*. Inhaled steroids have also been reported to be able to produce dysphonia, possibly as a result of myopathy of the phonatory muscles. It is assumed that the laryngeal lesion is directly related to the amount of corticosteroid passing through the vocal cords.

If long-term aerosol steroid therapy is inevitable, then beclomethasone dipropionate by inhalation is probably the agent of choice, with attention to possible candidiasis. However, a new aerosol preparation containing triamcinalone acetonide (Azmacort) has recently been introduced. It is claimed that this product delivers 90 to 95% of the metered dose to the airway, as compared to 40 to 60% for the beclomethasone system, and has a low incidence of oral candidiasis. Thus, it appears that aerosolized steroids can be substituted for oral steroids in most patients requiring less than 10 mg/day of prednisone, and a significant reduction in oral steroid dosage is possible in those requiring higher doses if aerosol administration is also used.

CROMOLYN SODIUM

Khellin, an extract of seeds from the Mediterranean plant *Ammi visnaga* Lam., has been known for centuries to have smooth muscle relaxing properties, and has found modest success in the treatment of bronchospasm. Unfortunately, this preparation produces too many side effects to be of clinical value. Studies in England during the 1960s identified a component active against allergic asthma, but with no bronchodilator property. It was introduced into the United States in 1973 under the name cromolyn sodium. The molecular structure of cromolyn sodium is unre-

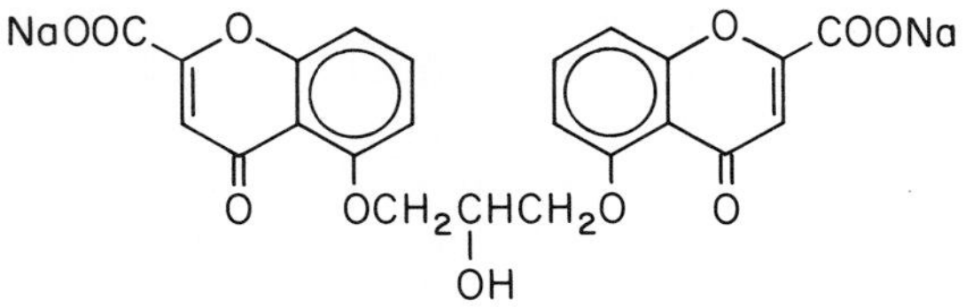

Figure 4-4. Molecular structure of cromolyn sodium.

lated to that of any other antiasthmatic drug; it is composed of two carboxychrome molecules bridged by an alkylene dioxy chain (Fig. 4-4).

Mechanism of Action

One of the first studies carried out with cromolyn sodium involved sensitized human lung tissue. In the presence of cromolyn, histamine and SRS-A release were decreased significantly on subsequent exposure to antigen. Apparently, the drug acts by stabilizing the mast cell membrane and preventing the release of mediators by preventing the calcium influx that triggers degranulation. Recently, it was demonstrated that cromolyn can induce the phosphorylation of a specific 78,000-dalton protein present in mast cells. It has been speculated that the phosphorylation of this protein may regulate a calcium "gating" mechanism (*i.e.*, Ca^{2+}-ATPase) associated with the entry of calcium into the cell.

The mast cell membrane receptor for cromolyn is specific, because the drug has no effect on basophils. Cromolyn cannot antagonize mediators that are already released. The drug has been found to be effective against both extrinsic atopic and intrinsic asthma, but cromolyn itself has no intrinsic anti-inflammatory or antihistaminic properties. Recent data suggest that cromolyn may also inhibit airway reactions by a direct effect on either bronchial irritant receptors or on smooth muscle.

It has been shown that cromolyn can prevent bronchospasm if administered prior to exposure of sensitized individuals to specific antigens. However, it is ineffective in reversing bronchospasm already produced in this manner. Therefore, cromolyn should only be administered prophylactically, because it has little efficacy once an asthmatic attack has commenced. Its mechanism of action has become synonymous with the phrase "antiallergic activity." The drug has been found to afford protection against recurring occupational asthma produced by platinum salts, piperazine, wood dusts, soldering fluxes, enzymes, toluene diisocyanate, and animal spasmogens. It has also been found to protect susceptible people from asthmatic attacks produced by exercise, hyperventilation, and aspirin.

Clinical Uses

Cromolyn appears to be most effective in children between the ages of 5 and 17 years. This is particularly advantageous if children in this age group have been maintained with glucocorticoids, because the dosage of steroid can be reduced or even eliminated. Various studies identify a variability in cromolyn's success rate, depending on the patient group. However, 50% of severe asthmatics may show some improvement.

Recommendations for patient selection include the following: patients maintained on more than 10 mg/day of prednisone or its equivalent; children and adolescents with reversible bronchospasm that is poorly controlled with conventional bronchodilators; patients with a predictable history of bronchospasm produced by allergens or industrial irritants; and individuals who develop postexercise asthma. Cromolyn therapy has no place in the treatment of those with acute bronschospasm or status asthmaticus, or of patients who suffer intermittent symptoms controllable by other means.

Because oral absorption of cromolyn is poor (lower than 0.5%), it is administered by inhalation. In fact, cromolyn is unique in that its administration involves inhalation of a dry powder. It is only effective in the treatment of asthma when applied in this topical manner. It is usually started on a dosage regimen (both for adults and children) of one capsule containing 20 mg of the drug and an equal amount of lactose (excipient) inhaled four times a day at spaced intervals. Considerable instruction may be necessary to facilitate the home therapy of some patients.

The powder blend is administered by means of a special turbo inhaler. Less than 4% of the drug will be deposited in the respiratory tract, with the remainder being swallowed. That which reaches the lung will be absorbed into the blood stream and excreted via the bile and urine within 4 hours. In view of its expense, cromolyn is usually reserved as an adjunct for use in moderately severe asthma that is not adequately controlled with bronchodilators.

Side Effects

Cromolyn is relatively free of side effects. Irritation of throat and airways, with reactive bronchospasm and exacerbation of status asthmaticus, can occur. The bronchospasm induced by the aerosol can be antagonized by administration of an aerosolized sympathomimetic bronchodilator 20 to 30 minutes prior to cromolyn. In a minority of patients hypersensitivity reactions can occur, which can range from skin rashes to potentially fatal anaphylaxis. Cromolyn is contraindicated in patients under 5 years of age, pregnant women, and those hypersensitive to the drug. Despite intensive work on antiallergy drugs of this type over the last 15 years, no satisfactory successors with oral efficacy have appeared on the market. However, it has recently been reported that a compound designated "Ro 22-3747" is being projected for clinical evaluation as an orally active antiallergic drug similar to cromolyn.

ANTICHOLINERGICS

At one time, extracts of *Atropa belladonna* (atropine) found some favor in the treatment of airway disease. For example, anticholinergic drugs were used in the 19th century in Europe in the treatment of asthma. Today, however, they have been replaced by the drugs mentioned previously, and are only used in patients who are resistant to the common drugs. Atropine is the prototypic competitive muscarinic blocker that can antagonize postganglionic parasympathetic nerve endings similar to those that emanate from the vagi and that supply the bronchiolar smooth muscle and mucous glands (see Fig. 4–1). The two most important effects of atropine are, therefore, antagonism of bronchoconstriction and reduction of secretions.

Disadvantages

Ostensibly, it would seem desirable to reduce secretions in the diseased airway. However, the use of atropine as a bronchodilator has been hampered because of fear that a net increase in mucous viscosity could occur. A recent study indicates that, although atropine can decrease sputum production in asthmatics, there is no measurable increase in viscosity. Atropine does decrease ciliary activity, however. Therefore, the potential for aggravating airway obstruction and the availability of superior agents have probably been the prime factors in atropine's diminishing popularity.

Ipratropium Bromide

Efforts are being directed at producing an atropinelike drug that acts selectively on bronchial smooth muscle. Ipratropium bromide is a new and potent anticholinergic bronchodilator currently undergoing clinical trials in the United States. This drug is a quaternary isopropyl-substituted derivative of atropine. It is administered by aerosol and appears to be an effective alternative to the use of traditional anticholinergics. It is marketed in Europe as a metered-dose aerosol containing 20 µg/puff administered in one to four puffs three or four times daily. Because of its route of administration, it exerts a selective bronchodilating effect in the larger airways. Its mechanism of action appears to be inhibition of acetylcholine-mediated increases in cGMP. Ipratropium appears to have little effect on ciliary activity, mucous secretion, sputum volume, or viscosity.

In clinical studies, ipratropium significantly increased 1- second forced expiratory volume (FEV_1) and other ventilatory parameters. The drug appears to be well tolerated following inhalation. Transient local effects were reported in 20 to 30% of patients, and included dry mouth, throat irritation, and a bad taste in the mouth. Systemic effects were rare and relatively minor. The consensus of opinion from the early clinical trials comparing ipratropium with β_2 sympathomimetics suggest that the drug is more effective in the treatment of chronic bronchitis than of chronic asthma. An additive effect between ipratropium and β_2 sympathomimetic aerosols has been reported in chronic bronchitis patients.

The role of anticholinergics in the treatment of bronchoconstrictive disorders remains to be clarified. If anticholinergics can be developed that do not lead to increased mucous viscosity, perhaps they may find use in chronic congestive states that involve a high degree of reflex cholinergic stimulation (*e.g.*, chronic bronchitis).

FUTURE DEVELOPMENTS

Several programs are presently underway for the development of alternative drugs for the treatment of asthma. For example, a number of new analogs of cromolyn are being evaluated, with particular emphasis on oral administration. In addition, because cannabis preparations have bronchodilator activity, attempts are being made to develop synthetic derivatives with selectivity for this effect relative to CNS actions. Perhaps the most exciting area of investigation involves the prostaglandins. Administration of PGEs (both PGE_1 and PGE_2) by aerosol to asthmatic patients indicates that these prostaglandins are more potent bronchodilators than isoproterenol administered by the same route, and that they have fewer significant effects on the cardiovascular system. However, these natural prostaglandins are not useful bronchodilator drugs because of upper airway irritation, reflex bronchoconstriction, potent cough induction, and a very short duration of action. Researchers are now synthesizing prostaglandin analogs with modifications aimed at overcoming these problems. An additional strategy is the development of structured analogs of spasmogenic prostaglandins and leukotrienes. The development of such competitive antagonists would appear to be highly desirable.

An *N*-isopropyl nortropine derivative of atropine currently under investigation in Europe appears to have a longer duration of action than isoproterenol and less drying of the mouth than atropine. If additional tests prove successful, this preparation may offer an effective alternative to current agents.

As indicated previously, calcium ions play a pivotal role in smooth muscle contraction. It has been suggested that agents that alter calcium movements might be valuable in asthma therapy. Calcium antagonists (*e.g.*, verapamil and nifedipine) are known to inhibit calcium ion influx selectively across the cell membrane and to suppress calcium-dependent smooth muscle excitation. These drugs are currently being investigated for their bronchodilating action. In addition, early studies suggest that calcium antagonists may prevent exercise-induced asthma. The protective effect presumably results from mast cells or from direct inhibition of tracheal smooth muscle contraction. However, other studies indicate that calcium blockers have little specific effect on immediate hypersensitivity reactions, and require relatively high doses. Hopefully, it may be possible to design calcium antagonists that will act preferentially on airway smooth muscle instead of on vascular tissues.

SELECTED REFERENCES

Becker, A. B., et al.: The bronchodilator effects and pharmocokinetics of caffeine in asthma. N. Engl. J. Med., 310:743, 1984.

Brittain, R. T., Dean, C. M., and Jack, D.: Sympathomimetic bronchodilator drugs. *In*: Widdicombe, J. G. (ed.): Respiratory Pharmacology, Section 104, International Encyclopedia of Pharmacology and Therapeutics, Oxford, Pergamon Press, 1981, pp. 613–655.

Christensson, P., Arborelius, M., and Lilja, B.: Salbutamol inhalation in chronic asthma bronchiale: Dose aerosol vs. jet nebuliser. Chest, 79:416, 1981.

Clark, S., and Newman, S.: Therapeutic aerosols. 2. Drugs available by the inhaled route. Thorax, 39:1, 1984.

Fredholm, B. B.: Are methylxanthine effects due to antagonism of endogenous adenosine? Trends Pharm. Sci., 1:129, 1980.

Harvey, J. E., et al.: Airway and metabolic responsiveness to intravenous salbutamol in asthma: Effect of regular inhaled salbutamol. Clin. Sci., 60:579, 1981.

Miller, M., et al.: Theophylline metabolism: Variation and genetics. Clin. Pharmacol. Ther., 35:170, 1984.

Newman, S. P., Pasia, D., and Clark, S. W.: How should a pressurized beta-adrenergic bronchodilator be inhaled? Eur. J. Resp. Dis., 62:3, 1981.

Pearlman, D. S.: Bronchial asthma: A perspective from childhood to adulthood. Am. J. Dis. Child., 138:459, 1984.

Snashall, P. D., Boother, F. A., and Sterling, G. M.: The effect of adrenoreceptor stimulation on the airways of normal and asthmatic man. Clin. Sci., 54:283, 1978.

Woenne, R., Kattan, M., and Levison, H.: Sodium cromoglycate-induced changes in the dose-response curve of inhaled methacholine and histamine in asthmatic children. Am. Rev. Resp. Dis., 119:927, 1979.

CHAPTER 5

Inhalation Therapy

OXYGEN

The lung is an absorptive organ, and thus provides access for drugs into the systemic circulation. Use of inhalation as a therapeutic mode of drug delivery is believed to have begun in 1794 with the publication of Considerations on the Medicinal Use and Production of Factitious Airs, by Beddaes. This treatise dealt specifically with oxygen therapy.

During this period in history, oxygen was enthusiastically applied for treatment of a wide diversity of maladies. Not surprisingly, many untoward effects resulted from such indiscriminate use. Even today, oxygen remains one of the most commonly used and misused drugs in hospital practice. In fact, oxygen is rarely thought of as a drug, with the result that it is used far less precisely than most other potent drugs.

There are several categories of abnormal respiratory function for which oxygen therapy is indicated. These classifications vary somewhat, depending on how much distinction between hypoxemia and hypoxia has been made by a particular author. For our needs, the term "hypoxia" will be used. Broadly defined, hypoxia will designate a deprivation of oxygen regardless of etiology or site. Various types of hypoxia and their description are summarized in Table 5–1.

The signs and symptoms of hypoxia are variable, and are dependent to a large degree on whether the deficit is acute or chronic and on the relative degree of hypoxia. Signs and symptoms associated with both acute and chronic hypoxia are presented in Table 5–2.

Therapeutic Uses of Normobaric Oxygen

Oxygen therapy of hypoxia usually does not correct the underlying problem but is employed as a stopgap measure until the basic defect has been corrected. The therapeutic uses of oxygen can be briefly described according to the various categories of hypoxia listed in Table 5-1. First, the use of 100% oxygen has now become an accepted part of high-altitude mountaineering, in which inspired air has an inadequate oxygen content. At the summit of Mount Everest (29,028 feet), for example, PO_2 is only

Table 5–1. Categories and Descriptions of Hypoxia

Category	Description
Inadequate O_2 content of inspired air	This may be caused either by a decrease in O_2 (%) in inspired air (presence of other gas) or by ambient pressure (high altitude)
Inadequate delivery of O_2 to alveoli	Normal O_2 tension with impaired ventilation; caused by airway obstruction, respiratory muscle weakness (disease or drugs), decreased respiratory drive (disease or drugs)
Inadequate oxygenation of blood	Normal O_2 tension and ventilation; alveolar-capillary diffusion block (acute and chronic pulmonary diseases)
Inadequate transport of O_2	Delivery failures: low cardiac output (shock), maldistribution of cardiac output (thrombosis, vasospasm); oxygenation failures: anemia, abnormal hemoglobin
Inadequate tissue uptake	High metabolic clearance (thyrotoxicosis, hyperpyrexia) or altered oxidative metabolism (cyanide poisoning)

50 torr (0.21% × 250 torr). Because of this scarcity of oxygen, it was not until 1978 that this mountain was successfully climbed by highly conditioned mountaineers without the aid of supplemental oxygen.

Second, in circumstances in which bronchoconstriction-induced obstruction is difficult to treat, hypoxia can be relieved with oxygen. However, inadequate delivery of oxygen to the alveoli does not always require therapy with oxygen; preferably, the cause of the hypoxia should be corrected. For example, obstruction of the airway can often be corrected by mechanical means. Furthermore, respiratory muscle failure or respiratory depression may merit artificial ventilation.

Third, inadequate oxygenation of blood because of abnormal pulmonary gas exchange constitutes the chief indication for oxygen. This usually occurs when hypoxia is the result of reduced diffusion of oxygen across the alveolar-capillary membrane or of ventilation-perfusion inequities. The diffusion of oxygen is reduced when anatomic changes occur, such as fibrosis or pulmonary edema. Oxygen inhalation can be of great benefit in these situations.

Oxygen therapy can also partially compensate for the decreased oxygenation of mixed arterial blood resulting from the perfusion of poorly ventilated alveoli. However, in certain situations, congenital or acquired shunts exist in which shunted blood is never exposed to respiratory gases. Oxygen therapy is less likely to be effective in such cases, because there is little room to increase the oxygen content of blood draining normal oxygen-containing alveoli.

Fourth, oxygen inhalation is useful in certain cases of inadequate transport of oxygen by the circulatory system. In carbon monoxide poisoning, for example, oxygen administration will result in a competitive displacement of carbon monoxide from hemoglobin. Increased oxygen dissolved in plasma will also help to protect tissues against hypoxia. Similar use of oxygen has been reported to be of value in the treatment of severe anemia. Oxygen has also been used effectively in certain cases of generalized (*e.g.*, shock) and localized (*e.g.*, coronary occlusion) circulatory deficiency to maintain adequate tension.

Miscellaneous uses of oxygen include the treatment of abdominal disorders (*e.g.*, intestinal obstruction, ileus, postoperative distention, pneumatosis intestinalis) and pulmonary conditions (*e.g.*, pneumothorax, air embolism) associated with nitrogen accumulation. Breathing 100% oxygen reduces the partial pressure of nitrogen in the alveoli to zero, and produces a concentration gradient for the gas out of tissue and blood into exhaled air. In anesthesia, oxygen is commonly used as a diluent for gaseous and volatile anesthetic agents.

Hyperbaric Oxygen Therapy

Most uses of oxygen do not require more than 1 atm of pressure. However, there are some conditions in which administration of hyperbaric tension may be helpful. Most such therapeutic situations are accomplished

Table 5–2. Possible Symptoms and Signs of Significant Hypoxia*

System Affected	Acute	Chronic
Respiratory	Breathlessness, tachypnea, hyperventilation, Cheyne-Stokes breathing, respiratory depression	Shortness of breath, dyspnea on effort, intolerance of increases in hypoxia (*e.g.*, from altitude)
Pulmonary	Pulmonary edema	Pulmonary hypertension
Cardiovascular	Increased cardiac output, vasodilation, palpitations, tachycardia, arrhythmias, hypotension, faintness, angina, acute cardiac failure	Cor pulmonale, decreased cardiac output, myocardial insufficiency, arrhythmias, unstable blood pressure
Central nervous	Euphoria, sleep disturbance, slurred speech, headache, impaired judgment, lassitude, inappropriate behavior, poor concentration, confusion, diplopia, papilledema, retinal hemorrhage, restlessness, lethargy, seizures, obtundation, coma, cerebral edema	Intellectual impairment, psychoneuroses, depression, paranoia, memory loss, insomnia, restlessness, irritability, tiredness, headache, papilledema
Neuromuscular	Fatigue, weakness, tremor, asterixis, hyperactive reflexes, incoordination	Myoclonic jerking, fatigue
Renal	Sodium retention, fluid retention	Edema, renal insufficiency
Other	Lactic acidosis, acidemia, cyanosis, diaphoresis, nausea, vomiting, cool extremities, shock	Polycythemia, vasodilation, plethora, clubbing, liver failure, tendency to venous thrombosis, poor tissue repair

*(From Ziment, I.: Respiratory Pharmacology, Philadelphia, W. B. Saunders, 1978, p. 457.)

in pressure chambers at approximately 2 to 3.5 atm. The primary objectives of hyperbaric oxygen therapy are to increase the volume of dissolved gas and to help push oxygen into the tissues.

The use of hyperbaric oxygen to treat decompression sickness (the bends) is perhaps its most important application. When divers breathe normal air under hyperbaric conditions (*e.g.*, 5 atm), nitrogen accumulates in tissues. If a diver surfaces too rapidly, nitrogen will effervesce and gas emboli will form in tissues that have been supersaturated with the gas. These minute bubbles are formed primarily in muscles, joints, bones, and nervous tissue, which results in severe musculoskeletal pains, visual and neurologic impairment, cerebral damage, and bone infarcts. Hyperbaric therapy recompresses the gas bubbles entrapped in tissues and reverses the symptoms described above. Hyperbaric therapy is followed by very slow decompression back to atmospheric pressure, much like the gradual loss of carbonation from a partially opened soft drink.

As mentioned above, oxygen therapy can be extremely beneficial in treating carbon monoxide poisoning. If a hyperbaric chamber is available, the use of 2 atm of oxygen for 30 to 90 minutes will result in even faster conversion of carboxyhemoglobin to oxyhemoglobin. Additional uses of hyperbaric oxygen include the intermittent treatment of gas gangrene produced by the anaerobic bacillus *Clostridium perfringens*, and circulatory disturbances such as stroke, peripheral arterial insufficiency, and compromised skin grafts. In rare circumstances, hyperbaric oxygen may be lifesaving in patients with severe anemia, hemorrhage, or hemolysis. In these situations the objective is to force as much oxygen as possible into the system. At one time, hyperbaric oxygen was considered to be of possible value in various forms of respiratory distress syndromes. Now, however, intensive respiratory care is considered to be more successful.

Oxygen Toxicity

When normobaric oxygen is administered to patients in concentrations exceeding the normal 21%, various side effects can appear, depending on the concentration, duration, and atmospheric pressure of exposure. Acute exposure to hyperoxia (21 to 100% oxygen) can produce characteristic toxic effects on the respiratory, cardiovascular, and pulmonary systems, the sinuses, the blood, and the eye. For example, with 100% oxygen at 1 atm, symptoms are likely to occur between 8 to 10 hours after exposure. These symptoms usually begin with tracheobronchial irritation, followed by coughing and dyspnea. It appears that patients may be exposed to 100% oxygen at 1 atm continuously for approximately 40 hours with minimal injury if the inspired oxygen is reduced to 40% thereafter.

Oxygen administration can lead to depression of respiratory drive, decreased transport of CO_2, and CO_2 narcosis. Cardiac output is decreased as a result of slight bradycardia and depression. In most areas of the body arteriolar constriction is produced by hyperoxia, except in the conjunctiva and in the pulmonary circulation in which vasodilation occurs. If oxygen replaces air in a body cavity during hyperoxia and is then absorbed, negative pressure is created, which can produce a sinus "vacuum headache."

Pulmonary responses range from nasal stuffiness and sore throat to alveolar and interstitial edema and fibrosis or atelectasis. Excess oxygen can also damage erythrocyte membrane integrity, leading to hemolysis. An area of particular concern is the exposure of premature infants to oxygen. Exposure of these neonates for hours or days to more than 40% oxygen can produce retrolental fibroplasia between the third and sixth weeks of life. This may regress, or may proceed to retinal detachment and blindness.

Hyperbaric 100% O_2 administration accelerates the development of the various syndromes of normobaric oxygen toxicity. Particular hazard is directed at the pulmonary and central nervous systems. When inspired oxygen becomes greater than 2 atm, central nervous system (CNS) toxicity is the first manifestation. Signs and symptoms include muscular twitching, nausea, vertigo, anxiety, paresthesias of the face and limbs and, finally, coma, convulsions, and death. Figure 5-1 presents a comparison of the times and onset of CNS and pulmonary toxicity in relation to duration of exposure and inspired oxygen pressure.

The probable mechanism of oxygen toxicity at the cellular level is the

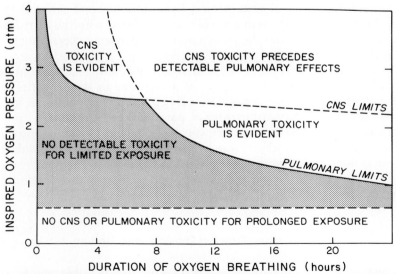

Figure 5-1. Comparison of onset of CNS and pulmonary toxicity in relation to duration of exposure and inspired oxygen pressure. (From Smith, T. C., Cooperman, L. H., and Wollman, H.: The therapeutic gases. *In* Goodman, A. G., Goodman, L. S., and Gilman, A. (eds.): Goodman and Gilman's The Pharmacological Basis of Therapeutics, 6th ed. New York, Macmillan, 1980. Copyright © 1980 by Macmillan Publishing Co., Inc.)

Table 5–3. Factors Modifying Oxygen Toxicity*

Hasten Onset or Increase Severity	Delay Onset or Decrease Severity
Adrenocortical hormones	Acclimatization to hypoxia
ACTH	Adrenergic blocking drugs
CO_2	Anesthesia
Convulsions	Antioxidants
Dexamethasone	Chlorpromazine
Dextroamphetamine	α-Aminobutyric acid
Disulfiram	Ganglionic blocking drugs
Epinephrine	Glutathione
Hyperthermia	Hypothermia
Insulin	Hypothyroidism
Norepinephrine	Immaturity
Paraquat	Intermittent exposure
Thyroid hormones	Reserpine
Vitamin E deficiency	Starvation
Exposure to x-rays	tris-(hydroxymethyl) aminomethane
	Vitamin E

*(Modified from Clark, J. M.: The toxicity of oxygen. Am. Rev. Resp. Dis., 110:40, 1974.)

generation of highly active free oxygen radicals. Oxygen radicals are thought to exert their lethal effect by generating single electron transfers within biologic systems that destabilize cell molecules and disrupt critical cell functions. At present, probable mechanisms of action involve the oxidation of sulfhydryl groups in enzymes, glutathione, and cofactors, and the peroxidations of unsaturated lipid double bonds in cell membranes. Lung injury from hyperoxia is also associated with the recruitment of activated neutrophils to the parenchyma, which may contribute to the pathology.

Because the lung is prone to oxidant injury, there is concern about a potential interaction between hyperoxia and toxins or drugs in the body when oxygen radicals are generated. Hyperoxia, for example, is known to potentiate the pulmonary toxicity of paraquat. Experimentally, protection against oxidant-induced injury can be achieved by the prophylactic administration of antioxidants (e.g., vitamin E) or of additional substrate (e.g., succinate, glutathione, and γ-aminobutyric acid). A more comprehensive list of factors that have been reported to modify the development of oxygen toxicity is shown is Table 5-3.

Other Gases: Carbon Dioxide and Helium

Carbon dioxide inhalation has been suggested as a therapeutic strategy in several common situations. However, it appears that for most of these conditions there are safer, more effective treatments. Situations in which carbon dioxide breathing has been purported to be efficacious include stimulation of respiration and coughing, hypocarbia, hiccups, cerebral vasodilation, and carbon monoxide poisoning (producing a shift to the right of the oxygen dissociation curve).

Helium is an inert gas with limited medical applications; its widest use is probably in deep diving. Helium is usually mixed with 20% oxygen for this purpose to replace nitrogen. Among its advantages are low density (one seventh that of nitrogen), which allows easier breathing of the mixture under hyperbaric conditions, and lower solubility in tissue lipids than nitrogen (one third). The result is less stress in breathing, with reduced decompression sickness and decompression time. Other characteristics of helium use include a high acoustic velocity (producing high-pitched voice distortion) and high thermal conductivity (body heat loss with severe shivering). Helium is also preferred at higher pressures because it has a lower narcotic potency than nitrogen, thus minimizing "rapture of the deep."

Clinical use of helium is restricted to selected cases of respiratory obstruction and pulmonary function testing. The use of helium in laryngeal or tracheal obstruction is based on the relationship of breathing energy to gas density. If obstruction is significant and the work of breathing air or oxygen is very high, mixtures of helium and oxygen may be respired with less effort. Helium's diagnostic use involves the introduction of a bolus of the gas and its subsequent dilution for calculations of diffusion capacity and functional capacity.

ANESTHETIC GASES AND VOLATILE LIQUIDS

Perhaps the most important group of therapeutic agents given by the pulmonary route are the anesthetic gases and volatile liquids. Early pharmacologic attempts to mitigate surgical pain included drugs such as ethanol and opium derivatives. Although the anesthetic and analgesic qualities of gases such as nitrous oxide and diethyl ether were known at the beginning of the 19th century, their use was primarily recreational—in carnival exhibitions and "ether frolics." The first attempt to demonstrate anesthetic efficacy was by Horace Wells in 1845. Unfortunately, his demonstration with nitrous oxide was a failure, and he died several years later, the victim of chloroform abuse. It was not until the successful demonstration of surgical anesthesia with ether in 1846 by William T. G. Morton that this procedure became a legitimate medical therapy, and ushered in a new era.

In the succeeding 140 years ether has been essentially discarded, while nitrous oxide continues to be used, and numerous new products have appeared. Between 1929 and 1959 cyclopropane was probably the most popular anesthetic. However, concern over cyclopropane's flammable nature stimulated research toward the development of a nonflammable agent, which resulted in the introduction of halothane in 1956. Halothane has become the most popular anesthetic in clinical practice. Most newer

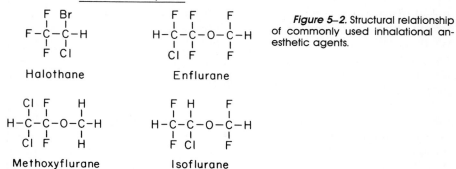

Figure 5–2. Structural relationship of commonly used inhalational anesthetic agents.

halogenated hydrocarbons are based on the halothane structure (Fig. 5-2).

Principles of Uptake, Distribution, and Elimination

General anesthesia produced by inhalational agents depends on the concentration (*i.e.*, partial pressure or tension) of the agent in the brain. Depth of anesthesia varies directly with the tension of the anesthetic agent in the brain, while the rates of induction and recovery depend on the rate of change of tension. The factors that determine the tension of an inhalational anesthetic in the arterial blood and brain are shown in Figure 5-3.

A number of theories have been proposed to explain the mechanism of action of gaseous anesthetics. These include stabilization of gas hydrate lattices, metabolic and electrolyte imbalances, and microtubule disorganization. However, the most popular model involves adsorption of the gas to nerve cell membranes, producing membrane expansion and destabilization of transmembrane pore structures. The result is inhibition of normal ionic fluxes, leading to nerve inexcitability.

As with any drug, the pharmacologic response to inhalation anesthetics is dose-dependent. Within the brain, regulation of an inhalation anesthetic's partial pressure is determined by its concentration in the blood. The tension of a gas in the blood, and therefore in the brain, is influenced by ventilatory rate and volume, perfusion of the lungs, and solubility of the agent in blood and body tissues.

The blood:gas coefficient of solubility can range from 12 for very soluble agents such as methoxyflurane to 0.47 for a relatively insoluble gas such as nitrous oxide (Table 5-4). Therefore, more highly blood-soluble anesthetic molecules will dissolve in the blood and body reservoirs (*e.g.*, muscle and fat) before producing a significant change in brain partial pressure. Figure 5-4 illustrates the inverse relationship between blood solubility of an anesthetic and the rate of increase of its arterial blood partial pressure.

In the case of highly soluble anesthetics such as methoxyflurane, anesthesia is achieved using the "overpressure" technique. With this method, the inspired tension is made much higher initially than the tension required in the brain for anesthesia. After achieving anesthesia, the inspired tension is progressively reduced to maintain a constant arterial and brain tension.

The factors mentioned above that affect gas uptake also regulate the rate of elimination of gaseous anesthetics, (*i.e.*, pulmonary ventilation, blood flow, and solubility in blood and tissue). When ventilation with nitrous oxide is terminated, for example, lung, blood, and high-flow visceral (brain) tensions of the gas decline rapidly. In such circumstances, the anesthetist or anesthesiologist almost has direct control of brain tension. Nitrous oxide will, of course, persist for a longer period of time in muscle and fat because these tissues have a lower blood flow. With an agent of very high solubility, a decrease of inspired tension produces only a very slow change of brain tension as a result of the "inertia" of the system.

Any volatile material, regardless of its route of administration, can be eliminated from the circulation via the lungs. The mechanism of elimination is simple diffusion, and is governed by lipid and blood solubility and partial pressure. The rate of elimination of volatile material from the circulation is directly related to pulmonary blood flow and respiratory rate. For example, in shock patients with reduced cardiac output, a decline

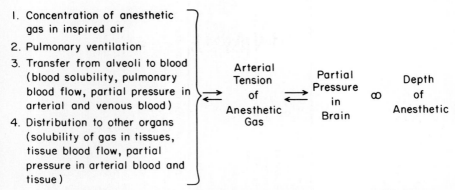

Figure 5-3. Factors determining the tension of an inhalational anesthetic in arterial blood and brain.

Table 5-4. Properties of Inhalation Anesthetics

Inhalation Anesthetic	Type	Blood: Gas Partition Coefficient (at 37° C)	Brain:Blood Partition Coefficient (at 37° C)	Minimum Alveolar Concentration (%)*
Nitrous oxide	Gas	0.47	1.1	105
Isoflurane	Volatile liquid	1.40	2.6	1.40
Enflurane	Volatile liquid	1.80	1.4	1.68
Halothane	Volatile liquid	2.30	2.9	0.75
Methoxyflurane	Volatile liquid	12.00	2.0	0.16

*Minimum alveolar concentration (MAC) is the anesthetic concentration at 1 atm that produces immobility in 50% of patients or animals exposed to a painful stimulus (*e.g.*, skin incision). It is an additive function. MAC decreases with age, hypothermia, pregnancy, hypotension, and use of central nervous system depressants.

in gaseous anesthetic-to-blood concentration to nonanesthetic levels will occur more slowly. These patients will, therefore, require more time to regain consciousness. Similarly, the use of a respiratory depressant such as an opiate analgesic for presurgical medication would be expected to prolong recovery from an anesthetic gas by reducing respiratory rate. Conversely, CO_2 is used during induction to increase ventilation and to increase blood flow to the brain.

The relative import of blood flow as compared to respiratory rate on the elimination of a volatile substance from the circulation depends on the blood solubility of that substance. Those substances that are relatively less blood-soluble (*e.g.*, nitrous oxide) are primarily influenced by cardiac output. They are excreted at roughly the rate at which blood delivers the molecules to the alveoli. Increasing cardiac output enhances their exposure to the alveoli, and increases their excretion in nearly a directly proportional manner. On the other hand, molecules that are relatively more blood-soluble (*e.g.*, halothane, ethyl alcohol) are less rapidly transferred from the pulmonary capillary blood to the alveoli. The rate of loss of these agents from the blood is, therefore, more dependent on respiratory rate than on cardiac output. The effect of increased respiratory rate is a shift in the partial pressure gradient of the substance in the direction of the alveoli, thereby encouraging the molecules to leave the blood.

Anesthetic gases and volatile liquids can also be eliminated, to varying degrees, by metabolism in the liver. For example, it has been reported that nearly 15% of halothane and 70% of methoxyflurane can be metabo-

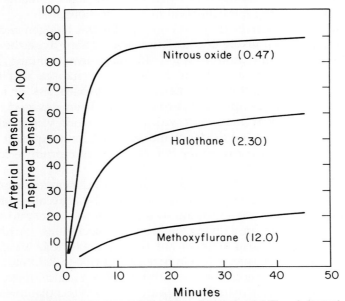

Figure 5–4. Inverse relationship of blood solubility of several anesthetics to the rate of increase of arterial blood partial pressure.

lized, producing various metabolites and ionized halogens. The significance of the hepatic metabolism of these halogenated anesthetics is not
necessarily the termination of their action, but rather the association of
hepatotoxicity with the metabolites formed therein. Specifically, halothane
can be metabolized to a chlorotrifluoroethyl free radical, which can react
with hepatic membrane components.

Volatile anesthetics can also influence the elimination of other drugs.
It is known, for example, that volatile anesthetics can decrease hepatic
blood flow either by myocardial depression (*e.g.*, enflurane, halothane),
direct splanchnic vasoconstriction (*e.g.*, cyclopropane, diethylether), or by
both (*e.g.*, methoxyflurane). Renal blood flow can also decrease during
general anesthesia. Consequently, hepatic metabolism and renal clearance
of certain drugs may be compromised during the period of anesthesia.

Effects of Gases and Volatile Liquids

Nitrous Oxide. The most commonly used anesthetic gas is nitrous
oxide. This weak anesthetic, when used alone at high concentrations,
produces hypoxia. Therefore, nitrous oxide is administered with at least
20% and preferably 30% oxygen. Nitrous oxide is used intermittently to
provide analgesia (possibly by opiate receptor agonism) for dental procedures and during the first stage of parturition. It does not produce skeletal
muscle relaxation. The principal use of nitrous oxide is in combination
with other anesthetic agents, thereby allowing the use of smaller doses of
the latter and reducing the likelihood of complications.

Nitrous oxide is nonexplosive and, unlike the halogenated volatile
anesthetics, is most unlikely to contribute to malignant hyperthermia (see
below). In high concentrations nitrous oxide may cause vomiting, hypoxia,
respiratory depression, and death. Postoperative nausea and vomiting
occur in approximately 15% of patients. An increased risk of renal and
hepatic diseases and peripheral neuropathy has been reported in dental
personnel who worked in areas in which nitrous oxide was used. Epidemiologic and experimental evidence indicate that long exposure to trace
concentrations of nitrous oxide may induce abortion or produce congenital
anomalies.

Halothane.   Smooth and rapid loss of consciousness and rapid awak-
ening from anesthesia account for the clinical popularity of halothane. In
addition, halothane is not an irritant to the respiratory tract and therefore
produces no increase in salivary or bronchial secretions. Furthermore,
pharyngeal and laryngeal reflexes are rapidly abolished. Nevertheless,
thiopental is routinely injected to induce sleep prior to halothane administration. Halothane is used for the entire range of surgical procedures.

Halothane can sensitize the myocardium to catecholamines, so the
heart could become more prone to arrhythmias. Conversely, cardiovascular depression occurs with increasing depth of anesthesia. Some bron-

chodilation has been reported with halothane, and may be related to its catecholamine-sensitizing effect. Halothane produces only moderate skeletal muscle relaxation; additional muscle relaxants (depolarizers) are thus used as adjuncts to maintain lighter levels of anesthesia. However, halothane augments the blocking effect of nondepolarizers (*e.g.*, *d*-tubocurarine), and their dosage should be reduced when used concomitantly.

Halothane administration has been associated with hepatic dysfunction, ranging from mild hepatitis to massive hepatic necrosis. The National Halothane Study reported massive hepatic necrosis in 0.27/10,000 patients receiving single administration of halothane and in 2.8/10,000 patients following multiple administrations. Severe halothane hepatotoxicity was recorded in 48 patients in a British Liver Unit over an 18-year period, and 38 of these cases proved fatal. The reaction is thus rare but dangerous. The median age of these patients was 57 years, the female to male ratio was 1.8:1, and 68% were judged to be obese. Those with drug allergies or eczema were more susceptible to the reaction, as were patients with more than one exposure to halothane.

A report from the British Committee on the Safety of Medicines on a series of 251 cases of jaundice following halothane administration showed that 75% of the patients had been exposed to this agent twice or more within 28 days. The mean interval between exposure and the onset of jaundice was 6.4 days in the multiple-exposure group, as compared with 11.4 days in the single-exposure group.

Three different mechanisms have been suggested for halothane-induced hepatotoxicity: the formation of an immunogenic metabolite; the formation of reductive metabolites that produce lipoperoxidation, covalent binding, or both; the induction of hepatic anoxia caused by the respiratory and cardiovascular depressant effects of the drug. Therefore, patients who appear to be at particular risk are those with recent exposure to halothane, hypoxic or ischemic liver, or prior liver disease, females, the obese, and those with previous allergies.

Another untoward effect occasionally seen in patients receiving halothane is malignant hyperthermia. This genetically linked hypermetabolic disorder is characterized by widespread skeletal muscular rigidity, elevated heat production by muscle, and a massive increase in oxygen consumption. Subsequent muscle damage can occur, and the hyperthermia may be fatal. Malignant hyperthermia may be triggered by most of the potent fat-soluble, inhalation anesthetics and by muscle relaxants (*e.g.*, succinylcholine).

Treatment includes rapid cooling, inhalation of 100% oxygen, and control of accompanying acidosis. The increased contraction of skeletal muscle appears to be the result of excessive release of calcium from the sarcoplasmic reticulum. For this reason, dantroline sodium has been used for prophylaxis and treatment because it appears to be able to decrease calcium release from the sarcoplasmic reticulum. Dantrolene should be administered intravenously as soon as malignant hyperthermia is evident, while oral administration may be necessary for several days to prevent recurrence.

Methoxyflurane. Methoxyflurane is the most potent of the inhalational anesthetics, and was introduced into clinical practice in the early 1960s (see Table 5-4). One of its main properties is its high lipid solubility, which contributes to its slow induction period (20 to 30 minutes), as a result of prolonged blood:tissue equilibration, and to its slow diffusion from fatty tissue, accounting for the persistence of analgesia and drowsiness following surgical anesthesia.

The effect of methoxyflurane on the cardiovascular system is similar to that of halothane, in that cardiovascular depression progresses with increasing depth of anesthesia. However, sensitization of the myocardium to catecholamines does not appear to be as great. Respiratory depression with methoxyflurane is slightly less than with halothane. In addition, because it does not irritate the respiratory tract, excess secretions and bronchoconstriction do not occur, thus minimizing the need for atropine-type premedications. When used alone, at a safe concentration, skeletal muscle relaxation is not significant. There is no evidence of direct hepatic toxicity although, as with other halogenated anesthetics, postoperative hepatic necrosis has been reported.

The most serious complication to methoxyflurane use is renal failure. This side effect was first reported in 1966, and it is now believed to be the result of its biotransformation. Methoxyflurane is metabolized to a greater extent than any other inhalation anesthetic agent, resulting in the liberation of significant amounts of fluoride and oxalic acid, both renal toxicants. The result is a toxic syndrome characterized by an inability to concentrate urine, with resulting polyuria; mortality rates in such patients may be as high as 20%. Obviously, administration of methoxyflurane to a patient with pre-existing renal damage is undesirable.

Because of the generation of unusually high plasma levels of fluoride (>40 μM), the use of methoxyflurane must be restricted to surgical procedures in which the duration of exposure does not exceed 4 hours, and, preferably, no more than 2. For this reason, and because it does not produce uterine relaxation, it is valued primarily for its analgesic potency during the first stage of labor. In this situation, small intermittent doses can reduce the accumulation of the toxic halogen.

Enflurane. Introduced into general clinical use in 1973 as a substitute for halothane, enflurane produces a smooth rapid induction (7 to 10 minutes), and emergence from anesthesia. Salivation and tracheobronchial secretions are not significantly stimulated, while laryngeal and pharyngeal reflexes are abolished early. As the depth of anesthesia increases, respiratory depression and hypotension become more probable. High P_{CO_2} levels can be obtained at deeper levels of anesthesia if ventilation is not supported. Cardiac output is not reduced as much as with halothane at low concentrations, so the hypotension is probably caused by decreased peripheral vascular resistance. Bradycardia is not a problem, and there is a reduced tendency to arrhythmias. Skeletal muscle relaxation is greater than with halothane, and may be adequate for intra-abdominal surgery. Therefore, if neuromuscular blocking agents are used to increase muscle relaxation, their dosage must be reduced. Enflurane also produces an enhancement of nondepolarizing neuromuscular blockers, although at a more gradual rate than halothane.

As with other halogenated volatile liquids, some evidence of hepatic impairment has been obtained. The incidence of necrosis, as well as mortality rate appears to be less with enflurane than with halothane. Nevertheless, it is suggested that in patients with a history of hepatotoxicity to related halogenated compounds (halothane or methoxyflurane), the use of enflurane should be avoided. Postoperative nausea and vomiting are less likely than with halothane or methoxyflurane (3 to 15%). Although enflurane is also metabolized, in part, to fluoride, plasma concentrations do not reach the threshold for renal toxicity, because approximately 80% of enflurane is expired unchanged.

It appears that anesthesia with enflurane in patients with renal disease will probably not be a problem if the depth and duration of anesthetic are not excessive. Enflurane use is associated with the appearance of self-limiting seizures of short duration. The clinical significance of this effect is controversial, because some authors have claimed no adverse clinical consequence while others have recommended that enflurane not be used in patients with a history of seizures.

Enflurane can be used for the induction and maintenance of general anesthesia, because a good depth of anesthesia can be achieved rapidly and smoothly with fewer side effects than with halothane or methoxyflurane. However, deep anesthesia is associated with respiratory depression; thus, as the depth of anesthesia increases, assisted or controlled ventilation may be required. Increased seizure activity is associated with inspired concentrations of 3%. Deep levels of anesthesia with enflurane should also be avoided during labor, because uterine smooth muscle becomes relaxed.

Isoflurane. This pungent-smelling volatile anesthetic is an isomer of enflurane, but has a more rapid induction and recovery from anesthesia. In contradistinction to other halogenated agents, myocardial function is well maintained, with concentrations ranging from 1 to 2% minimum alveolar concentration (MAC). Blood pressure does decrease with dose but returns toward normal with surgical stimulation. Isoflurane does not sensitize the myocardium to catecholamines, salivation and tracheobronchial secretions are not a problem, and pharyngeal and laryngeal reflexes are readily obtunded.

Isoflurane can produce significant respiratory depression, characterized by decreased tidal volume and unchanged respiratory rate. Muscle relaxation is adequate for intra-abdominal operations at normal levels of anesthesia. Complete muscle paralysis is attained with small doses of muscle relaxants. The dose of depolarizing neuromuscular blocking drugs used concomitantly should be decreased by one third.

Summary. The ideal inhalation anesthetic would possess, among other things, a rapid onset of sleep with analgesia, decreased visceral reflexes, and skeletal muscle relaxation, all with a minimum of side effects. Unfortunately, no such agent is known. The anesthetics used today vary in their relative efficacy to achieve these various effects. Halothane, for example, produces good narcosis. However, opiates or nitrous oxide is used concurrently to achieve analgesia, while muscle relaxation and visceral reflexes are managed with other drugs. The volatile anesthetics are almost always administered in combination with 40 to 70 vol % nitrous oxide, which reduces the quantity of volatile anesthetic required. A summary of the major inhalation anesthetic effects is shown in Table 5-5.

Although inhalation anesthetics are an indispensable group of drugs, they are among the most dangerous drugs approved for use. The slopes of the dose-response curves for inhalational anesthetics are steep, which means that the margin of safety in their use is small. In fact, the therapeutic indices for these drugs range from approximately 2 to 4. It has been estimated that more than 1000 deaths annually in North America result from the use of inhalation anesthetics or from an anesthesia-related error.

LOCAL ANESTHETICS

General Considerations

Local anesthetics are used topically for diagnostic procedures, such as endoscopy, to depress the cough or gag reflex by blocking sensory nerve function. Their mechanism of action is believed to be twofold in nature. First, the principal process involves attachment of the cationic form to a phospholipid receptor on the internal axoplasmic membrane. This complex prevents ion flux and propagation of nerve impulses, and stabilizes the membrane. Second, the un-ionized form is believed to occupy a critical volume of the nerve membrane, leading to conformational distortion of the protein(s) necessary for ion flux and depolarization. The relative contribution of each is dependent on the pK_a of the anesthetic in question. An anesthetic with a pK_a in the range of 7.6 to 9.0 will act primarily via the former mechanism, while an anesthetic with a very low pK_a (3.5) will act via the latter.

Absorption and toxicity from topical use of local anesthetic agents differ according to site of application. In general, absorption occurs most rapidly following intratracheal administration and more slowly following intranasal instillation. These differences are caused, in part, by the inherent variations in vascularity of the different anatomic sites, and by the properties of the pharmaceutic preparations utilized for topical anes-

Table 5–5. Summary of Inhalation Anesthetic Effects

System	Agent				
	Halothane	Enflurane	Isoflurane	Methoxyflurane	Nitrous Oxide
Cardiovascular					
Cardiac output	→	→	→	→	↑ (Low); ↓ (high)
Peripheral resistance					↑ (Low); ↓ (high)
Catecholamine sensitization	Yes	Minor	No	Less than halothane	No
Respiratory					
Tidal volume	→	→	→	→	Minor
Respiratory rate	←	←	←	←	
Brain					
Metabolic rate	→	→	→	→	→
Cerebral blood flow (increased intracranial pressure)	←	←	←	←	Least ↑
EEG suppression	Yes	Yes	Yes	Yes	
Spike-and-wave pattern	Yes	Yes			
Skeletal Muscle					
Relaxation	Some	Greatest	Adequate	Some	No
Malignant hyperthermia	Yes	Yes	Yes	Yes	Unlikely
Uterine Muscle					
Relaxation	Yes	Yes	Yes	No	Minor
Kidney					
Renal blood flow	→	→	→	→	Minor
Glomerular filtration rate	→	→	→	→	Minor
Renal failure				Main limitation*	

*When more than 1 MAC is used for more than 2 hours, the likelihood of fluoride accumulation becomes significant.

thesia. Rapid absorption from the tracheobronchial tree, for example, is undoubtedly related not only to the vascularity of this area but also to the use of anesthetic sprays, which tend to disperse the anesthetic solution over a wide surface area. On the other hand, local anesthetic agents that are commonly applied to mucous membranes in the nasal cavity are done so in the form of an ointment or gel, which tends to delay vascular absorption.

Tetracaine appears to be absorbed very rapidly from the trachea. In fact, its LD_{50} is similar for intratracheal and intravenous administration. The significance of this is revealed by the fact that several deaths have followed the use of intratracheal tetracaine. The principal signs of local anesthetic toxicity include CNS excitation (including convulsions), and systemic hypotension secondary to peripheral vasodilation and myocardial depression. For topical use, it is recommended that one third of the established maximum safe dosage used for infiltration anesthesia be employed.

Only the major agents will be considered in this section. They are classified as being used primarily for local anesthesia of the nasopharyngeal-laryngeal or tracheobronchial regions.

Nasopharyngeal-laryngeal Area. A popular local anesthetic for this region is benzocaine. Because it has a low pK_a, the un-ionized form easily penetrates the mucosa. Benzocaine is available in numerous forms, including aerosol spray, liquid, ointment, and gel. It is valuable for anesthetizing the nose or throat prior to nasotracheal intubation. Piperocaine is also useful for nasal anesthesia when used as a 1% jelly on endotracheal tubes. Lidocaine is often sprayed onto a nasal mucosa and onto the back of the pharynx as a 10% solution.

Many clinicians consider cocaine to be a popular anesthetic for bronchoscopic procedures. It is both safe and effective, and has no antimicrobial potency, which is an important consideration if specimens are to be cultured for bacteria and fungi. Aerosol administration of a 10% solution can anesthetize the nasopharynx-larynx, and a 4% solution can then be used for the segmental bronchi.

In individuals allergic to one of the above agents dyclonine may serve as an alternative, because it has a different structural basis (ketone) and less cross antigenicity. The potency of dyclonine is comparable to that of cocaine with an onset of 10 minutes and a duration of action of up to 1 hour. It is usually given as a 0.5% gargle for anesthetizing the throat, and it does have antimicrobial potency.

Tracheobronchial Region. The most popular and widely used local agent for topical anesthesia of the respiratory tract, used for both laryngoscopy and bronchoscopy, is lidocaine. Its application basically involves three steps: spraying of a 4% solution into the oropharynx; transmucosal block of superior laryngeal nerves by swabbing of the piriform sinuses; and spraying of the epiglottis with a 2% solution.

Subsequent does of lidocaine are often given to maintain suppression of cough and gag reflexes. This can have potential toxicologic significance, because entry of lidocaine into the systemic circulation has been documented following topical administration during bronchoscopic procedures. In some cases, serum concentrations exceeding 3 μg/ml have been reported. This is considered to be a high therapeutic concentration, and patients with cardiac disease may be at particular risk.

SELECTED REFERENCES

Brown, B. R.: Pharmacology of general anesthesia. *In* Goth, A. (ed.): Medical pharmacology. St. Louis, C. V. Mosby, 1984, pp. 385–407.

Grogono, A. W., and Seltzer, J. L: A guide to drug interactions in anesthetic practice. Drugs, 19:279, 1980.

Marshall, B. E., and Wollman, H.: General anesthetics. *In*: Gilman, A. G., Goodman, L. S., and Gilman, L. (eds.): Goodman and Gilman's The Pharmacological Basis of Therapeutics, New York, Macmillan, 1980, pp. 276–292.

Smith, T. C., Cooperman, L. H., and Wollman, H.: The therapeutic gases. *In*: Gilman, A. G., Goodman, L. S., and Gilman, L. (eds.): Goodman and Gilman's The Pharmacological Basis of Therapeutics, New York, Macmillan, 1980, pp. 321–338.

Trevar, A. J., and Miller, R. D.: General anesthetics. *In*: Katzung, B. G. (ed.): Basic and Clinical Pharmacology, Los Altos, Lange Medical Publications, 1982, pp. 255–261.

Versey, M P.: Epidemiological studies of the occupational hazards of anesthesia. Anesthesia, 33:430, 1978.

CHAPTER 6

Upper Respiratory Infections

PATHOGENICITY

General Considerations

It has been estimated that the general practitioner will see between 700 and 1000 patients with respiratory diseases each year. The most prevalent forms of respiratory ailment are the viral-induced common cold and flu, which are primarily self-limiting upper respiratory infections. The demarcation between the upper and lower respiratory tracts is the transition from terminal bronchioles into respiratory bronchioles. Susceptibility to viral infection depends on the integrity of respiratory tract defense mechanisms, such as filtration, physical entrapment (by mucus), and chemical inactivation by immunologic mechanisms.

The common cold is caused by a number of different viruses. Approximately 80% of colds are caused by the RNA rhinovirus, of which 90 serotypes have been identified, and about 15% are caused by the RNA coronavirus. These viruses usually enter the body through the nostrils or conjunctiva via self-contamination. It has been reported that, in adults with a cold, 40% had viruses on their hands, but only 8% expelled viruses in coughs or sneezes.

The flu is caused by various influenza viruses, classified into three main groups (A, B, and C), depending on their nucleoprotein composition. Influenza A is the principal cause of pandemics, while the B type is associated with the milder winter epidemics. Changes in the antigenic makeup of these viruses takes place continuously, and accounts for localized outbreaks. For example, the Hong Kong flu epidemic of 1968–1969 resulted in 51 million reported cases and 80,000 deaths in the United States.

The onset of the common cold is usually sudden, following a 2- to 4-day incubation period. The characteristic symptoms include sore throat, sneezing, runny nose, watery eyes, mild fever, aches and pains, nasal congestion and coughing. Complications of the common cold can also include sinusitis, otitis media, and respiratory tract bacterial infections, including tracheitis, bronchitis, bronchiolitis, and lobular pneumonia.

The symptoms of systemic disturbance may be even more severe with influenza. Malaise, muscular pain, fever and, occasionally, nausea and vomiting, may be experienced.

Self-Treatment

A substantial proportion of the population uses nonprescription over-the-counter (OTC) remedies to self-treat the symptoms of these maladies. Yearly sales of OTC cold medications alone exceed one billion dollars. Because there is little essential difference between the average prescription preparation and the popular OTC products, the latter will be given the most emphasis in this review. Unfortunately, most cough and cold medications have been found by government panels of experts to lack effectiveness. In addition, many contain four or more ingredients, thereby subjecting the user to a greater potential risk of adverse effects. Among the more questionable preparations is Nyquil, which contains 50-proof alcohol selling for almost 11 dollars a fifth.

There are five principal components of cold and flu preparations aimed at relieving the major symptoms of these viral infections: sympathomimetic amines, antitussives, expectorants, anticholinergics, and antipyretic-analgesics. They are available in an almost limitless variety of combinations, and the number of products on the market will probably increase in the near future. This is because the FDA has listed ten ingredients that can be sold in OTC products, that were previously available only by prescription. Antihistamines are also often included in cold and flu preparations, and the merits of this strategy will be assessed. Because of its popularity, vitamin C will also be discussed.

DECONGESTANT SYMPATHOMIMETIC AMINES

The mucous membrane of the nose is a common site for irritation and infection because it is the first tissue contacted by all respirable materials. Lysis of the virus-bearing host cells during common cold attacks destroys upper respiratory membranes, resulting in local inflammation caused by mediator release, with attendant capillary dilation leading to interstitial edema, and with a reflex increase in mucous secretion and mucosal permeability. Edema of the nasal mucosa can be particularly bothersome, because this area has a rich vascular supply that forms subepithelial plexuses of arterioles. The large volume of blood that can be diverted into these plexuses during inflammation can produce significant engorgement of the nasal mucosa. Therefore, both capillary dilation and the mucus contribute to nasal congestion. When the nasal mucosa is significantly congested, the passageway through the turbinated airway becomes a major factor in air flow resistance.

Sympathomimetic compounds are used topically and orally because of their vasoconstrictor property (α-receptor activation), which produces a physiologic antagonism of vasodilation. By causing vasoconstriction, pore size is reduced and fluid loss from the capillaries is decreased. There are two major classes of α-adrenergic decongestant drugs: β-phenylethylamine derivatives, and imidazoline derivatives. Most OTC preparations have traditionally contained β-phenylethylamine derivatives (*e.g.*, phenylephrine, phenylpropanolamine, pseudoephedrine, ephedrine). However, the longer acting imidazoline derivatives are increasing in popularity, and their use will probably become predominant (Table 6–1).

Topical Administration

The advantage of topical administration of sympathomimetic drugs to the nasal mucosa is a rapid onset of action at the affected site. The classic decongestant constituent of topical cold preparations has been phenylephrine (Fig. 6-1). Phenylephrine is a short-acting derivative of epinephrine, possessing only one hydroxyl group on the benzene ring. Its most effective use is via nasal instillation for topical treatment of mucosal congestion. However, its use for more than 3 to 5 days should be discouraged, because "rebound" congestion can occur. In this condition, the mucosal vessels become less sensitive to α-receptor activation, with a resultant vasodilation. Complete withdrawal of the vasoconstrictor results in spontaneous reversal of the "rebound" congestion, usually within 48 hours. The "rebound" effect is more common with the chronic use of stronger concentrations: at a concentration of 0.25%, phenylephrine has been seldom reported to produce this condition.

Imidazoline derivatives, including naphazoline, tetrahydrozoline, oxymetazoline, and xylometazoline, are more potent, longer acting (8 to 12 hours) α-sympathomimetic decongestants than phenylephrine (4 hours). They are usually administered topically as drops or spray, with the latter being more effective. They are also used in ophthalmic preparations to decrease redness. Their structures are significantly different from that of phenylephrine (Fig. 6-1). Naphazoline and oxymetazoline have been reported to be more likely to produce nasal mucosa irritation. However, this is generally compensated for by their longer duration of action, and they are a good choice as topical nasal decongestants.

Imidazoline derivatives should be used with care in the treatment of nasal congestion in small children and infants. Increased absorption of naphazoline and tetrahydrozoline is a potential source of pediatric toxicity and has been reported to produce severe CNS depression, leading to coma. This can best be avoided by the proper administration of nasal sprays (head in an upright position) or by the use of drops. Finally, the marketing of "adult" and "pediatric" strength topical decongestant drugs is considered unjustified by some experts because of the similarity of adult

Table 6–1. Sympathetic Vasoconstrictor Drugs Used as Nasal Decongestants

Drug	Predominant Route of Administration	Usual Dosage Form	Comments
Imidazoline Derivatives			
Naphazoline	Topical	0.05% solution	Not recommended for children under 6 yr old
Oxymetazoline	Topical	0.05% solution	Somewhat longer acting, with milder side effects
Xylometazoline	Topical	0.05–0.1% solution	Long-lasting, with generally mild and infrequent side effects
Tetrahydrozoline	Topical	0.05% solution	Marked tendency to cause rebound congestion, with no advantages
β-Phenylethylamine Derivatives			
Phenylephrine	Topical	0.125–1% solution	Oldest topical preparation, with short duration of action
Phenylpropanolamine	Oral	25- and 50-mg tablets	Most widely used oral product; properties similar to those of ephedrine, without CNS stimulation
Pseudoephedrine	Oral	30- and 60-mg tablets	Stereoisomer of ephedrine; less CNS stimulation and hypertension
Propylhexedrine	Inhalation	250-mg/dose nasal inhaler	Use should be discouraged in children; extracted and injected IV by drug abusers.

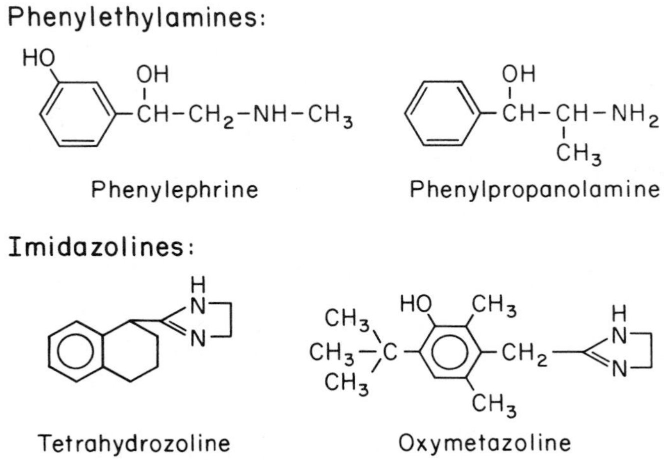

Phenylethylamines:

Phenylephrine   Phenylpropanolamine

Imidazolines:

Tetrahydrozoline   Oxymetazoline

Figure 6–1. Comparison of structural formulas of commonly used sympatho-mimetic decongestants.

and child nasal mucosa. Nevertheless, the availability of an alternative dose form may be beneficial to those with sensitive nasal mucosa.

Nasal decongestants can also be found in inhalers. Examples of effective ingredients are propylhexedrine and 1-desoxyephedrine. Inhalers may be less effective for some people, because it may be difficult to deliver the medication in this form into a congested nose.

Oral Administration

Although the oral route of administration affords a potentially longer duration of action, with no nasal irritation or associated "rebound" congestion, oral sympathomimetics are, nevertheless, not considered to be as effective or safe as topical preparations. In fact, oral vasoconstrictor drugs rarely do much to relieve nasal stuffiness, mainly because of inadequate dosage (more than 40 mg is required), nonlocalized deposition (resulting in a lower concentration of the drug at the receptor site), and disseminated distribution (which permits interaction of the drug with various receptors, leading to side effects). Because the vasculature of the nasal mucosa is not more sensitive to adrenergic drugs than other blood vessels, oral doses large enough to produce nasal decongestion can be expected to constrict other vascular beds.

A potential side effect produced by oral preparations containing the popular phenylpropanolamine is elevated blood pressure, which repre-sents a hazard for the 22 million Americans with high blood pressure. One recent study indicated that, when single doses of phenylpropanolam-ine (85-mg capsule or 50-mg sustained-release capsule) were given to a group of healthy young adults, the supine diastolic blood pressure rose to 100 mm Hg or more in a significant number of volunteers. However, OTC preparations do not contain this amount of phenylpropanolamine. Several cases of severe hypertensive crises following ingestion of phenylpropanolamine at doses found in many new prescription preparations have also been described in the literature. In general, however, these drugs do not raise blood pressure when the usual low dose of decongestant is used.

Ephedrine has been a traditional decongestant ingredient in certain cold remedies. Unfortunately, ephedrine has numerous drawbacks, including CNS stimulation, potential aggravation of blood pressure, short duration of action, and tolerance. There seems little to recommend this drug as a decongestant today. However, a stereoisomer, pseudoephedrine, would appear to be the most desirable oral preparation, because it has fewer cardiovascular and CNS effects than phenylpropanolamine and ephedrine, respectively.

Patients 60 years of age or older appear to be particularly susceptible to adverse reactions associated with OTC oral sympathomimetic use, especially because those in this age group tend to have disorders that are aggravated by additional adrenergic activity, such as hypertension, hyperthyroidism, diabetes mellitus, ischemic heart disease, angina, advanced arteriosclerosis, increased intraocular pressure, and prostatic hypertrophy. Habituation and toxic psychosis have also been reported following long-term high-dose therapy.

Elderly patients are also most likely to experience drug interactions with sympathomimetics, because they are often likely to take β-adrenergic blockers or monoamine oxidase (MAO) inhibitors concurrently. Severe hypertensive reactions may, for example, occur when sympathomimetics are given to patients receiving MAO inhibitors.

Mixtures

Mixtures containing decongestants with antihistamines, antibiotics, analgesics, or anticholinergics are available. However, there is no satisfactory evidence to substantiate claims that any of the available mixtures is more effective than a single-entity drug if nasal decongestion is the only desired effect. If relief from other symptoms is also sought, then the appropriate additional ingredient should be taken separately.

Visual hallucinations and dystonic reactions have been reported as rare side effects of decongestant-antihistamine mixtures. For example, in a trial of pseudoephedrine, triprolidine, and placebo in the treatment of respiratory symptoms associated with otitis media, 6% of children had to be withdrawn because of side effects such as irritability, dizziness, general malaise, and nightmares. Decongestant-antihistamine mixtures are second only to antibiotics in prescriptions issued to children. They are often given for their presumed sedative effects, but there is no evidence that these mixtures are more effective then placebo in treating sleep disturbances in children with respiratory symptoms.

Adult respiratory distress syndrome may develop after relatively small overdoses of drugs containing phenylpropanolanine. Postmortem examination of a 15-year-old girl 31 hours after intentional consumption of eight to nine capsules of a mixture of phenylpropanolanine (50 mg) and belladonna alkaloids (0.2 mg) revealed congested lungs with increased capillary wall permeability.

ANTITUSSIVES

Effects of Coughing

Coughing is a protective physiologic reflex that serves to clear the respiratory tract of irritants and the product of that irritation, mucus. The cough reflex mechanism involves afferent sensory activation of the "cough control center" in the base of the brain (medulla), which, through appropriate cholinergic pathways, produces rapid intake of air and closure of the epiglottis, contraction of chest and abdominal muscle while the bronchi are constricting, and release of the epiglottis with an air velocity that can approach 500 miles/hour.

Coughing generally removes the mucus that accumulates during periods of mucosal irritation. In performing this function the cough plays an important productive role that should not be suppressed. Sometimes, however, dry nonproductive coughs occur, which become part of a vicious cycle of cough-irritation-cough. In such cases suppression of coughing can bring substantial pain relief to the patient without compromising an important defense mechanism. However, the frequency with which cough preparations are prescribed and purchased indicates that, in actual practice, such products are used much more extensively than can be defended.

According to a 1975 report, there were more prescription products available for treatment of cough than for any other symptoms accompanying a cold. Because the cough has both peripheral and central components, there are several possible sites for drug action. Many OTC cough lozenges contain benzocaine, for example, which can act as a topical anesthetic on the inflamed mucous membrane. For minor irritations these products are often sufficient. However, more severe attacks of coughing usually require products with more substantial centrally acting properties.

Centrally Acting Antitussives

The yardstick against which all other antitussive agents are evaluated is the opium alkaloid codeine, first isolated in 1832. Subjective and objective tests have shown codeine to be an effective antitussive drug. It is undoubtedly the most prescribed antitussive in the United States, and is available in numerous proprietary preparations in a wide range of doses that usually do not produce significant side effects in healthy adults. Depending on the preparation, a prescription may or may not be required. For example, if codeine is present in a concentration not higher than 200 mg/100 ml, no prescription is necessary (schedule V). Preparations containing up to 1.8 g/100 ml, however, may be ordered by regular prescription (schedule III).

Codeine is not recommended for infants younger than 6 months old, however, because of their inadequate development of their glucuronidation detoxification mechanism. In doses required for cough suppression, the addictive liability associated with codeine is low. An equal antitussive dose of codeine has been reported to possess only 5% the psychologic effect of morphine. Additional comparisons to morphine indicate that codeine has 25% of the depressant effect on respiration, less chance of causing nausea, vomiting, and constipation, and less chance of causing release and bronchospasm in asthmatics. Nevertheless, abuse can lead to severe psychologic or physical dependence, if severe enough. The usual adult dose is 10 to 30 mg in a single dose, which may be repeated after 3 to 4 hours.

A compound structurally related to the opiates but not a narcotic agent is dextromethorphan. This (+) isomer is the most widely used cough suppressant in the United States. It is claimed that dextromethorphan has three major advantages over codeine, having less abuse potential, fewer respiratory depressive effects, and lower gastrointestinal inhibition. In addition, there is no effect on sputum or ciliary activity. The consensus is that dextromethorphan is a weaker (50%) but safer antitussive than codeine. Like codeine, dextromethorphan acts by depressing the cough center. Receptor binding sites localized in brain stem areas such as the floor of the fourth ventricle have been identified for cough suppressant agents such as dextromethorphan. Dextromethorphan should not be used for persistent cough such as that which occurs with smoking, asthma, or emphysema, or when cough is accompanied by excessive secretions. The usual adult dose is 15 to 30 mg every 4 to 6 hours.

Side effects, including dizziness, headache, nausea, and vomiting, have been reported following doses of 60 mg or more, but are infrequent with the usual oral dose. As with other morphine derivatives, dextromethorphan should be used with caution in patients receiving MAO inhibitors, because the drug-drug interaction can produce CNS depression and death.

Although there are numerous other antitussives on the market, none offers any significant advantage over codeine or dextromethorphan, and some probably have little more than placebo value. Hopefully, with pressure from the FDA, these less efficacious products will be withdrawn from the market.

In summary, codeine would appear to be the most effective and economical narcotic antitussive available, while dextromethorphan is the best nonnarcotic cough suppressant with less relative potency but certain advantages. For most patients, dextromethorphan in single-entity products is the most appropriate treatment of severe dry unproductive cough.

EXPECTORANTS

Manufacturers claim that expectorants help to relieve coughing by thinning out the respiratory tract fluids so that they can be more easily expelled. Their purported mechanism of action involves stimulation of vagal efferents (via the vomiting center), which innervate bronchial glands. This is highly theoretic, however, because there is no unequivocal evidence demonstrating efficacy of the dozen or so ingredients that have been alleged to perform this function. In fact, the FDA advisory panel on cough and cold remedies concluded, in their 1976 report, that no expectorant qualified for classification in category I (generally recognized as effective). It is also interesting to note the pharmacologic contradiction of formulations having cough facilitators and suppressants in the same preparation, as is often the case.

For an expectorant to be effective it should decrease mucous viscosity, increase mucous clearance, and improve ventilation. Clinical studies have generally shown no detectable decrease in sputum viscosity or increase in sputum volume with the use of the expectorant agents. Ideally, an effective expectorant should facilitate the removal of excess bronchial fluid rather than promote its secretion. Because the available expectorant products have essentially no efficacy, there appears to be no reason to prescribe or encourage their use.

Most of these agents have an emetic action resulting from vagal stimulation, and it has been suggested that subemetic doses of these drugs cause expectoration rather than vomiting. Glyceryl guaiacolate, guaifenesin, and guaiacol glyceryl ether are the most prevalent expectorants found in OTC as well as in prescription preparations. Chronic therapy with large doses appear to be necessary for any observable effect. Most investigators have not found guaifenesin to be useful, and it has been reported that glyceryl guaiacolate can interfere with biochemical diagnostic tests based on the use of 5-hydroxyindolacetic acid and vanillylmandelic acid.

Other less frequently employed expectorants include ammonium chloride, terpin hydrate, sodium citrate, and iodides. These agents merit little consideration, other than to indicate that large doses of ammonium chloride can produce metabolic acidosis, which is particularly hazardous in patients with improperly functioning lungs, liver, or kidneys, and that the combination of terpin hydrate with cough suppressant drugs such as codeine and dextromethorphan has no logical basis.

At present, at least with regard to the common cold, humidification of room air and adequate fluid intake (6 to 8 glasses daily) may be the most effective therapeutic measures that can be taken to mobilize respiratory tract secretions.

ANTICHOLINERGICS

These agents are usually atropine or scopolamine, or a derivative thereof. They are often included in combination preparations for their drying effect on mucous secretions. As mentioned previously, both smooth muscle and secretory glands of the airway receive vagal innervation and contain muscarinic receptors. Competitive blockade of these receptors with atropinelike drugs would be expected to decrease glandular secretion and to relax bronchial smooth muscle. However, the FDA advisory panel did not find any anticholinergic generally recognized as effective.

The use of anticholinergic drugs seems unnecessary. If a drying effect is necessary, an antihistamine with anticholinergic properties (such as diphenhydramine) would probably be more effective. Furthermore, the addition of an anticholinergic agent seems to be equally inappropriate in a combination product already containing an antihistamine, because an additional drying effect is unlikely to be significant and may, in fact, be deleterious.

By including these anticholinergic agents in multidrug formulations containing expectorants that supposedly act to increase secretions, many drug companies have succeeded in producing "irrational" products. Not only do many of the individual ingredients counteract each other, they also significantly increase the risk of adverse reactions without providing additional therapeutic benefit.

ANALGESIC–ANTIPYRETIC–ANTI-INFLAMMATORY AGENTS

Certain combination cold remedies contain either aspirin or acetaminophen; the rationale for their inclusion is to relieve the associated aches and pains, headache, and fever. Arguments can be made for or against their inclusion. For example, if fever is slight it may provide some pyrogenic antiviral effect, and should not be antagonized. On the other hand, the general malaise that often accompanies a cold or the flu can often be relieved by these agents. If either aspirin or acetaminophen is purchased, a generic or house brand should be selected, because the consumer will save approximately 50 to 70% of the cost of brand name products.

Comparison

Aspirin and acetaminophen are approximately equipotent in terms of both their antipyretic and analgesic activities. However, in cases in which pain is largely caused by tissue inflammation, aspirin is the superior product. The explanation for this divergence in activity may be related to variations in cyclooxygenase sensitivity. It has been suggested that cyclooxygenase from both peripheral tissues and the CNS are sensitive to aspirin, while only that from the CNS is affected by acetaminophen.

Side Effects

The most common side effect of aspirin is gastric irritation. The exact mechanism is unknown, but a widely accepted theory is that of acid back diffusion. In essence, aspirin is believed to facilitate the diffusion of hydrogen ions back into the gastric mucosa, producing pain and bleeding. Aspirin is also known to interfere with normal blood clotting by inhibiting platelet aggregation, and by reducing plasma prothrombin levels at high doses (>6 g/day).

Aspirin use is contraindicated in diabetics receiving oral hypoglycemic drugs (sulfonylureas) because aspirin can displace them from plasma protein-binding sites, thus increasing their effective free concentration. Other drugs that may interact with aspirin include warfarin anticoagulants, sulfinpyrazone, probenecid, and spironolactone.

Two types of hypersensitivity reactions can occur with aspirin use. The first is characterized by asthmalike symptoms, and may be related to a shunting of arachidonic acid through the leukotriene pathway when aspirin inhibits cyclooxygenase. The second is dermal in nature, involving reactions such as edema, rashes, and hives.

The use of aspirin in children with influenza (flu) or with chickenpox has been strongly linked with the subsequent occurrence of Reye's syndrome, an often fatal disease. Physicians and parents should avoid using aspirin or salicylate (aspirin)-containing medicine in children 18 years old or younger for treatment of chickenpox or during the flu season.

Acetaminophen has fewer side effects than aspirin. However, there have been isolated reports of hepatotoxicity caused by low-dose acetaminophen use. This is a warning sign, because acetaminophen has been classified as a predictable hepatotoxin—that is, if large doses (*e.g.,* 10 g) are given to animals or intentionally ingested by humans, liver damage inevitably follows. The mechanism of hepatotoxicity involves the formation of *N*-acetylimidoquinone via cytochrome P_{450}. This toxic metabolite is highly reactive and can combine directly (covalent bonding) with hepatocyte macromolecules, leading to necrosis. The seriousness of potential hepatotoxicity merits advising patients against long-term ingestion of the drug at doses exceeding those normally recommended. Alcoholics are particularly sensitive to the hepatotoxic effects of acetaminophen.

Aspirin is still considered by most people to be the drug of choice for relieving the pain associated with the common cold. However, there are some data suggesting that the relief achieved through its anti-inflammatory effect may be at the expense of other cold-related factors. For example, it has been reported that aspirin can increase viral shedding and, therefore, increase the likelihood of reinfection. Another study indicates that aspirin blocks the effect of interferon (see below). The anti-inflammatory effect may also be responsible for an immunosuppressant effect, such as that of glucocorticoids, which could enhance viral replication.

ANTIHISTAMINES

The presence of antihistamines in cold preparations has become a controversial subject. Originally hailed as "the cure" for the common cold in the 1940s, there remains little theoretic justification for their use in the treatment of the common cold. Clinical studies indicate no evidence that antihistamine usage either relieves the symptoms of a cold or shortens the duration of the illness, primarily because histamine release does not appear to be a significant factor contributing to cold symptoms, which are the product of virus-induced cell lysis.

The efficacy of antihistamines in reducing rhinorrhea is undoubtedly a consequence of their inherent anticholinergic properties. However, this drying effect can be a disadvantage with cold sufferers because a more irritating cough can result. In addition, because antihistamines can thicken bronchial secretions, they act in opposition to expectorants that supposedly thin out secretions. Furthermore, a study has also failed to confirm the effectiveness of antihistamine-decongestant combinations in preventing otitis media.

It has been recommended that the label of cold preparations indicate that antihistamines are "for the temporary relief of runny nose, sneezing, itching of the nose or throat, and itchy and watery eyes as may occur in hay fever, but not for the relief of nasal symptoms, such as stopped-up nose, nasal stuffiness, or clogged-up nose." The antihistamines will be described in more detail in Chapter 7.

VITAMIN C

In 1970, Linus Pauling published his controversial book, *Vitamin C and the Common Cold*. Since that time, numerous studies have been carried out attempting to assess the pharmacologic efficacy of this antioxidant. On the basis of results obtained thus far, vitamin C does not appear to possess significant virucidal, anti-inflammatory, or antihistaminic properties.

The most positive, if not unequivocal, results obtained with vitamin C relate to improvement of host immune function. There is some evidence suggesting an elevation of serum antibody levels in subjects receiving chronic vitamin C. However, more emphatic results indicate that vitamin C is associated with increased phagocyte activity, increased macrophage mobility, increased interferon levels and chemotaxis in neutrophils, and stimulation of epithelial basement membrane formation.

The use of large doses of vitamin C is associated with several important pharmacologic principles. First, the absorption of vitamin C from the gastrointestinal tract requires a saturable, active transport system. At doses ranging up to approximately 180 mg/day, the absorption of ascorbic acid is 80 to 90% complete, but at a dose of 1.5 g, for example, only 50% is absorbed. This clearly indicates less bioavailability, a greater likelihood of local gastrointestinal disturbances, and less cost effectiveness.

In addition, large doses on the order of 1 g are less metabolized, and up to 80 to 90% of the unchanged weak acid may be excreted unchanged in the urine. This can result in acidification of the urine, with an increased likelihood of precipitation of renal stones. In people taking unusually high doses of ascorbic acid (*e.g.*, 9 g) there is the additional possibility of increased formation of oxalic acid from ascorbic acid because of metabolic shunting. Therefore, the formation of renal calculi becomes a distinct possibility.

In conclusion, the available evidence at this time indicates the following: (1) vitamin C appears to have little effect on the incidence of the common cold, but may reduce the severity of its symptoms; (2) the effects produced by vitamin C are variable and dependent on sex, virus type, and host age; and (3) a 200- to 300-mg daily intake of vitamin C is unlikely to be harmful, although large 1-gram or more doses present some hazards.

VACCINES AND INTERFERON

Developing a vaccine against the common cold is fraught with several difficulties— for example, the fact that natural immunity to the common cold is so rare casts doubt on the production of an effective vaccine. In addition, because 90 or so serotypes of the prevalent rhinovirus exist, there is an obvious immunologic challenge.

Interferons were discovered in 1957, and have been found to have a wide range of biochemical functions, including the modulation of immune responsiveness and cellular control. Interferons are soluble proteinaceous materials rapidly produced by the host cell (see further on) following viral infection. They appear to act by binding to receptors on cell surfaces followed by inducing the synthesis of enzymes that inhibit viral replication. In humans, three different types have been described: lymphocyte (α), fibroblast (β) and type II or immune (γ).

Interferon is believed to play a significant role in host defense against not only the common cold but against cancer and other infections as well. However, the few clinical studies that have been carried out have not demonstrated much success, which could conceivably be a result of poor dosing and drug delivery, because early studies were limited by the availability of only small amounts. Another problem has been extreme cost. In one study, interferon was administered by nasal spray 1 day prior and 3 days following exposure to a cold virus, and these two sprays cost a total of 14 dollars. Attempts to obtain large amounts of interferon inexpensively appear to be most promising with cloning of the interferon gene in *Escherichia coli*. Presumably, genetic engineering will make interferon(s) more readily available in the future.

SELECTED REFERENCES

Block, M.: (1984). Acetaminophen hepatotoxicity. Ann. Rev. Med., 35:577, 1984.
Kaufman, J., et al.: Over-The-Counter Pills That Don't Work. New York, Pantheon Books, 1983, pp. 33–66.
Koda-Kimble, M. A.: Therapeutic and toxic potential of over-the-counter agents. *In* Katzung, B. G. (ed.): Basic and Clinical Pharmacology, Los Altos, Lange Medical Publications, 1982, pp. 738–741.
Po, A.: Non-Prescription Drugs, Oxford, Blackwell Scientific Publications, 1982, pp. 234–302.
Wolfe, S.: Pills That Don't Work, New York, Warner Books, 1980, pp. 29–42, 87–88, 112, 133–134.

CHAPTER 7

Immunopharmacology of the Lung

IMMUNE SYSTEM

Three major host defense systems exist to protect the lung against inhaled foreign particles and noxious gases: mechanical barriers, clearing mechanisms, and the immune system. Mechanical barriers and clearing mechanisms have been dealt with previously; this chapter will describe the immune system. Although the immune system defends the body against airborne substances, it can sometimes respond in a manner that is, ironically, injurious to the host.

Immune responses are generally classified as nonspecific or specific. A nonspecific response in the lung would involve the phagocytosis of a bacterium or virus by an alveolar macrophage. The ability of the macrophage to phagocytize bacteria is influenced by the composition of the bacterial capsule. Because phagocytosis involves passage through a membrane, nonpolar capsules are accommodated more easily. Conversely, more polar capsules (*e.g., Streptococcus pneumoniae*) are not dealt with as effectively by the macrophages. Nonspecific responses occur in everyone, and are greatly augmented after activation of a specific response.

Components

Specific immune responses are characterized by humoral-mediated and cell-mediated effector systems. Two groups of cells within the lymphoid tissue of the lung accomplish these tasks. These lymphocytes are referred to as B and T cells, respectively, originate in the bone marrow, and are found in lymph nodes, submucosal nodules, bronchus-associated lymphoid tissue, and in interstitial spaces.

For the purpose of the discussion here, emphasis will be placed on the B cells. These lymphocytes contain specific receptors on their cell membranes, which can combine with specific portions of antigen molecules known as antigenic determinants. Binding of antigen to B-cell receptors elicits the synthesis of specialized proteins called immunoglobins (antibodies; Fig. 7–1). Activation of B cells requires the interplay of growth and differentiation factors as well as lymphokines.

Although the lung is not generally regarded as a lymphoid organ, it is an important tissue source of antibody. There are four immunoglobulins found in the respiratory tract: IgA, which is the predominant form and is found along the airway, IgM, found at low concentration along the airway, IgG, synthesized locally in the lower airway because of serum transudation, and IgE, synthesized locally in the nasopharynx and airway. IgE is implicated as the mediator of allergic rhinitis, conjunctivitis, extrinsic asthma, and anaphylaxis.

There are five major processes by which immunoglobulins function to protect the airway against invading antigens: opsonization, the combining of antibodies with capsule protein to decrease polarity and produce more efficient phagocytosis; precipitation, the formation of antigen-antibody complexes, with subsequent insoluble aggregates; agglutination, which is similar to precipitation, with a "clumping" of cells; toxin neutralization, the binding of antibody to a toxin to produce an alteration in its active site; and complement activation, formation of active cascade fragments by antigen-antibody complex.

HAY FEVER

"Hay fever" is a generic term that refers to a multitude of windborne pollen-mediated allergies. Although there is debate over the origin of the phrase, it probably reflects a cause-and-effect association between exposure to harvested wheat and to the feeling of warmth that ensues (*i.e.*, histamine-induced vasodilation). Hay fever is primarily characterized by seasonal attacks of rhinitis and sneezing. It is estimated that approximately 13 million Americans suffer from allergic rhinitis. Other discomforts associated with hay fever include stuffy nose, conjunctivitis, wheezing, coughing, and itching throat and ears. Initially, allergic episodes may be confused with the common cold.

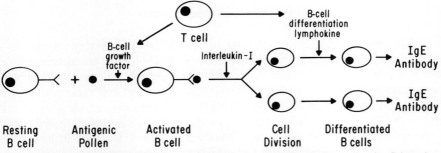

Figure 7–1. Simplified diagram of pollen-induced antibody formation by B lymphocytes.

Table 7–1. Comparison of Symptoms and Treatment of the Common Cold and Hay Fever Allergy

| Symptom | Major Mediator | Intensity | | Therapy |
		Allergy	*Cold*	
Runny nose	Histamine	+ + +	+	Antihistamine
Watery eyes	Histamine	+ +	+	Antihistamine
Congestion	Histamine	+	+ +	Sympathomimetic, decongestant, antihistamine
Aches and pains	Prostaglandins	0	+	Aspirin
Fever	Prostaglandins	0	+	Acetaminophen, aspirin
Headache	Prostaglandins	0	+	Acetaminophen, aspirin
Sneezing	Reflex	+ +	+	No direct treatment
Coughing	Reflex	+	+ +	Topical, central

There are quantitative and qualitative differences between the common cold and hay fever, which should be taken into consideration when therapy is appropriate. For example, sneezing is more likely to occur with "hay fever" than with a cold, because large pollen molecules are preferentially deposited in the nasal passages and upper pharynx, in distinction to smaller viruses. In these areas, inflammation-induced mechanical and chemical stimulation of sensory nerves produces sneezing. A brief comparison of the major symptoms of the common cold and hay fever is shown in Table 7–1.

Hay fever symptoms reflect localized involvement of the immune system. As noted above, the immune system is a host defense mechanism that evolved to protect the lung against inhaled foreign particles. However, an immune response can result in pathologic reactions and tissue injury. The immunologic reaction involved with hay fever is classified as type I (immediate hypersensitivity). Because competency for immunoglobin production is under genetic control, the risk of developing hay fever is an inherited predisposition.

Biochemical Mechanism

After an individual has become sensitized (by primary exposure) to a pollen, the IgE molecules that were formed and released by differentiated B-cell lymphocytes function as ligands, and attach to mast cells in the respiratory tract and circulating basophils. The mast cell receptor for IgE has been identified as a two-component complex, one protein of which binds the IgE. Repeated exposure to an antigen results in more rapid production of large numbers of antibodies. Serum IgE levels in hay fever patients rise, therefore, as the pollen season progresses.

The creation of IgE antibodies has also endowed them with the ability to bind to the antigenic determinant that first stimulated their creation. In essence, thus, the immune system has produced a new group of receptors for the antigen, which are attached in series to effector cells (*e.g.*, mast cells). Subsequent exposure to the antigen results in an antigen-antibody interaction on the surface of mast cells that alters membrane permeability and elicits degranulation, with mediator release.

To initiate the release process, it is necessary for a divalent antigen to cross link two IgE molecules (Fig. 7–2). A simplified description of the steps involved in mediator release include the following: increased influx of calcium (opening of "calcium gates") caused by activation of a serine esterase, phospholipid methylation, and perhaps a membrane protein; calcium activation of phospholipase A_2 leading to leukotriene formation; and mediator release.

Autacoids released as a result of mast cell degranulation include histamine, SRS-A, eosinophil chemotactic factor of anaphylaxis (ECF-A), and platelet activating factor (PAF). In humans, histamine interacts with receptors (H_1), producing stimulation of exocrine glands, dilation of blood vessels, with increased permeability, and bronchoconstriction. Although the predominant effect of histamine on airway smooth muscle in most species is contraction, it has been demonstrated that the airway of some species contain H_2 receptors that mediate airway relaxation. The availability and activity of H_1 and H_2 receptors varies both among species and also within a given species with their location within the lung. However, H_2 receptors do not appear to play a significant role in human airways, which probably explains why cimetidine (H_2-blocker) has little effect on airway responsiveness. Histamine appears to be responsible for most symptoms of hay fever. Although the role of SRS-A in hay fever is unclear, it is believed to be a significant factor in producing bronchoconstriction in

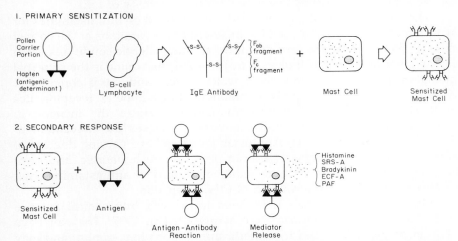

Figure 7–2. Sequence of principal events involved in antigen-antibody interaction leading to mediator release.

extrinsic asthma. The specific contributions, if any, of ECF-A and PAF to hay fever remain to be delineated.

Treatment

There are basically two approaches to the treatment of hay fever: desensitization and drug therapy. The therapeutic procedure known as desensitization or immunotherapy is widely established in the practice of medicine. There are over 3000 allergy specialists in the United States. The regimen of desensitization developed largely as a result of empiric observations that injections of allergen extracts could, in certain cases, reduce the severity of a patient's symptoms to seasonal allergies. However, the concept of allergy was not involved in these original applications but, rather, the notion that pollen contained toxins that could provide immunity to such patients with a vaccine composed of pollen extract. As our knowledge of allergy developed, the process of inoculation became known as desensitization.

Desensitization implies the administration of graduated doses of an allergen over a several-month period of time, with diminishing responses. In practice, the success achieved is variable, and depends on the patient and on the allergen in question. According to the FDA, many allergen extracts used for injection lack evidence of effectiveness. In fact, of the hundreds of pollen extracts, the Panel on Review of Allergenic Extracts found only four to be effective. When effective, the mechanism appears to involve an interaction between IgG and IgE immunoglobins. It has been suggested that the process of desensitization may result in the formation of IgG antibodies that either compete with mast cell-bound IgE for the allergen or possibly interfere with the synthesis of IgE.

The vast majority of hay fever sufferers depend on antihistamines for symptomatic relief. When used in single-entity preparations at the correct dosage, these agents are very useful for genuine allergic conditions, such as hay fever or hives. As indicated in Table 7–1, histamine is the principal mediator, producing runny nose, watery eyes, and nasal congestion. Antihistamines act as competitive inhibitors at histamine H_1 receptor sites in these areas. This competitive antagonism reduces the increase in capillary wall permeability and, therefore, decreases the movement of fluid from blood into tissue. Antihistamines also have varying degrees of affinity for other receptors, which can produce anticholinergic, antipruritic, and sedative effects. It is the sedative property of antihistamines that has been utilized in the formation of OTC sleep aids.

Over 50 antihistamines have been introduced into clinical practice since the first antihistamines were synthesized in 1937. They all have pharmacologic actions and therapeutic applications in common, and may be discussed in general terms. Knowledge of the chemical classification of antihistamines is useful, because a patient may fail to respond to one particular antihistamine, and an alternative produced from another chemical group may be necessary. Most antihistamines are substituted ethylamines and are classified on the basis of their structure (Fig. 7–3; Table 7–2).

Antihistamines are usually taken orally, and effects appear within 15 to 30 minutes. Most have a duration of action of approximately 3 to 4 hours, and are principally metabolized in the liver. A few of the longer acting sustained-release preparations (*e.g.*, triprolidine) may be effective for as long as 24 hours. In seasonal rhinitis, antihistamines are most effective at the beginning of the season when pollen counts are low. As

Table 7–2. Chemical Classification of Selected Antihistamines

Drug	Main Clinical Uses and Side Effects
Ethanolamines	
Bromodiphenhydramine	General antihistamine, with sedative and anticholinergic effects
Carbinoxamine	General antihistamine, with less sedative and other side effects
Diphenhydramine	General antihistamine, with sedative and anticholinergic effects; agent of choice for administration by injection
Phenyltoloxamine	Main use is for rhinitis; principal side effect is sedation
Ethylenediamines	
Chloromethapyrilene	General antihistamine, with little sedative properties, but can produce nausea
Methapyrilene	General antihistamine that can be used topically or parenterally; dizziness and headache have been reported side effects
Pyrilamine	Used mainly for rhinitis; produces little sedation and few side effects
Thenyldiamine	Used mainly for rhinitis as nasal solution or spray; slight sedation
Tripelennamine	General antihistamine producing slight sedation and possible nausea
Alkylamines	
Brompheniramine	Used mainly for rhinitis; can produce drowsiness
Chlorpheniramine	Most widely used OTC antihistamine; produces slight drowsiness
Dexbrompheniramine	Twice as potent as brompheniramine
Dexchlorpheniramine	Twice as potent as chlorpheniramine
Dimethindene	Long-acting general anesthetic
Pyrrobutamine	Long-acting general antihistamine, with minimal side effects
Triprolidine	Long-acting potent antihistamine, with minimal side effects
Piperazine	
Hydroxyzine	Antihistamine reported useful in asthma; principal side effect is drowsiness
Phenothiazine	
Promethazine	Antihistamine with antiemetic property; principal side effect is drowsiness

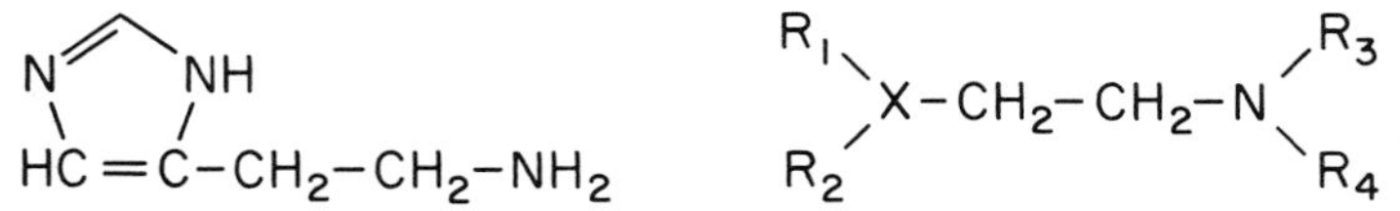

$$\begin{array}{c} N \overset{\displaystyle{\nearrow}}{\diagdown} NH \\ N \diagdown \quad \diagup \\ HC = C - CH_2 - CH_2 - NH_2 \end{array}$$

$$\begin{array}{c} R_1 \diagdown \quad \diagup R_3 \\ X - CH_2 - CH_2 - N \\ R_2 \diagup \quad \diagdown R_4 \end{array}$$

Histamine   Basic Antihistamine Structure

Figure 7–3. Comparison of histamine and antihistamine structures.

the concentration of pollen in the inspired air increases, these drugs become less effective. For unknown reasons, the effectiveness or toxicity of a specific drug seems to depend on the individual patient.

The use of a single effective antihistamine ingredient, such as chlorpheniramine maleate or brompheniramine maleate, both available in inexpensive generic versions, is probably the preferred treatment for hay fever. Timed-release forms have been advocated for the treatment of hay fever, but their action is unpredictable and the additional cost is unnecessary.

The most common side effect produced by antihistamines is drowsiness; the extent of the drowsiness produced depends on the particular antihistamine. Relatively speaking, ethanolamine derivatives and phenothiazines produce the most drowsiness. This side effect has been exploited in the development of OTC sleep aids (*e.g.,* methapyrilene). Obviously, simultaneous use of other depressant drugs such as alcohol can be a dangerous combination, and should be avoided.

Antihistamines also have varying degrees of anticholinergic effects; the most important one relevant to the respiratory system is excessive drying of the respiratory tract. This results in the development of viscid bronchial secretions, which are more difficult to expectorate. A second feature that further compromises patients with excessive lower respiratory tract secretion is impairment of mucokinesis. Therefore, antihistamines are not recommended for the treatment of bronchial asthma in cases in which accumulation of mucus is a problem. Additional peripheral anticholinergic effects include blurred vision and tachycardia. Frequent side effects also involve the digestive tract, and include nausea, vomiting, diarrhea, and loss of appetite. Such side effects may be reduced by giving the drug with meals.

A new drug approved by the FDA for the treatment of hay fever is sodium cromoglycate for intranasal use (Nasalcrom). Although presently requiring a prescription, it has been sold over the counter for years in the United Kingdom. The dose for adults and for children 6 years and older is one spray in each nostril three to six times daily at regular intervals. Treatment is most effective if started prior to expected contact with the offending allergen.

However, clinical studies indicate that intranasal beclomethasone diproprionate (BDP) is more effective than intransal sodium cromoglycate in the treatment of seasonal rhinitis. BDP has been widely used for many years as topical intranasal therapy for the management of both seasonal and perennial rhinitis. It has been found to be highly effective, and has not been shown to produce any abnormal histologic changes on the nasal mucosa after long-term use. Pressurized and aqueous preparations are equally effective when administered daily in divided doses of 200 μg each, and this dose produces no change in adrenal function. The most common side effect of BDP is nasal irritation.

ALLERGIC ASTHMA

As mentioned in Chapter 6, asthmatic episodes can be precipitated in susceptible individuals by exposure to specific antigens. The terms "extrinsic" and "atopic" are often used to designate that segment of the population that has a genetic predisposition to antigenic factors. The clinical history of asthmatic patients is generally one of multiple allergies, including hay fever, food, and eczema.

Mechanism

The pathophysiology associated with allergic asthma is the result of mediator release from sensitized lung tissue. There are many putative mediators, but the factor responsible for clinical asthma is unknown. The small degree of protection afforded by H_1 blockers in asthma clearly indicate the importance of chemical mediators other than histamine. Possible mediators of current interest are members of the prostanoid family, such as leukotrienes, prostaglandins, and thromboxane. As described previously, the leukotrienes (C_4, D_4, and E_4) are believed to comprise SRS-A and, therefore, play a major role in this disease. In humans, leukotrienes are potent bronchoconstrictors and contribute to the edema and mucous hypersecretion that occurs in asthma.

Experiments in the guinea pig with intravenously administered leukotriene D_4 indicate that tracheal contraction is directly mediated, while bronchoconstriction occurs via direct and indirect mechanisms. The latter is a consequence of thromboxane A_2 generation. Aerosol administration of leukotriene D_4 induces bronchoconstriction only by a direct mechanism. The importance of leukotriene generation by way of the lipooxygenase pathway in allergic asthma probably explains why cyclooxygenase inhibitors (e.g., aspirin, indomethacin) have not proved to be clinically efficacious in asthma. In fact, studies indicate that cyclooxygenase inhibitors can induce asthma-like symptoms in nonasthmatics, presumably by redirecting arachidonic acid metabolism through the lipoxygenase pathway. A great deal of effort in the pharmaceutic industry is now being directed toward the development of leukotriene antagonists for use in asthma.

Classification

Four types of allergic reactions are associated with immunologic diseases of the lungs. The type I immune response is the basic reaction seen with allergic respiratory tract diseases such as hay fever and extrinsic asthma. This immune response is characterized by a quick onset of symptoms, becoming maximal in 10 to 20 minutes. Resolution generally occurs in 1 to 2 hours. This immediate type of response also characterizes the more extreme anaphylactic reaction. Type I responses are produced by antigen-IgE interactions on the surface of mast cells.

The Cyclic Nucleotide System

Cyclic AMP has been known for approximately 20 years to play a central role in most secretory systems, including mediator release. However, its exact role still remains to be elucidated. It is known that the potency of β-adrenergic agonists in inhibiting mediator release correlates well with their ability to increase cAMP in certain preparations (*e.g.*, human leukocytes, mast cells, basophils).

As mentioned previously (Chap. 4), a poor correlation exists between the concentration of methylxanthines needed to produce *in vivo* therapeutic effects and *in vitro* inhibition of phosphodiesterase activity. Similarly, attempts to demonstrate that methylxanthines inhibit mediator release *in vitro* have not been successful. Recently, however, it has been reported that pharmacologic concentrations of theophylline can block a group of adenosine receptors that normally potentiate antigen-induced mediator release and bronchoconstriction.

DRUG ALLERGY

Allergic reactions to drugs occur relatively infrequently. It has been estimated that less than 10% of all adverse reactions have an allergic basis. The most serious manifestation of drug allergy involving the lung is anaphylaxis, and the greatest offender by far is penicillin and its semisynthetic derivatives.

Mechanism

An allergic response requires the presence of a macromolecule that is identified by the body as an antigen and that promotes the formation of antibodies. Antigens are usually large molecules with molecular weight in the tens of thousands. Because drugs generally have a molecular weight of only a few hundred daltons, a different process must be involved.

Low-molecular-weight chemicals that are incomplete antigens are called haptens. To develop full antigenic expression, an irreversible conjugation of the hapten to a high-molecular-weight molecule, such as a protein, must take place by covalent bonding. Such a complex may now become antigenic. As a rule, parent drugs themselves do not react with protein, but first undergo metabolism to a more chemically reactive metabolite.

Penicillin produces a number of haptenic determinants during the course of its metabolism; the major determinant is the penicilloyl moiety formed by opening of the β-lactam ring (Fig. 7–4). Minor determinants include penicilloate and penicillamine. Major and minor determinant refer to the frequency with which antibodies to these haptens are formed, and not to the severity of the allergic reaction. Antigenic determinants can also be formed *in vitro* as a result of the breakdown of penicillin and of the formation of penicilloyl polymers. Penicillin is particularly prone to undergo degradation in the presence of carbohydrates and certain metal ions, such as iron.

Anaphylaxis

Anaphylactic reactions to penicillin are thought to occur in about 1 to 5/10,000 patient courses of treatment, and have been estimated to cause 400 to 800 deaths annually in the United States. This immediate type I response is characterized by bronchospasm, mucous membrane congestion, angioedema, and cardiovascular collapse. The anaphylactic response is mediated by IgE antibodies. An anaphylactic response most often follows injection of penicillin, although oral, intradermal, and even respiratory administration have produced anaphylaxis in susceptible patients.

Avoidance of an anaphylactic response is most easily achieved by

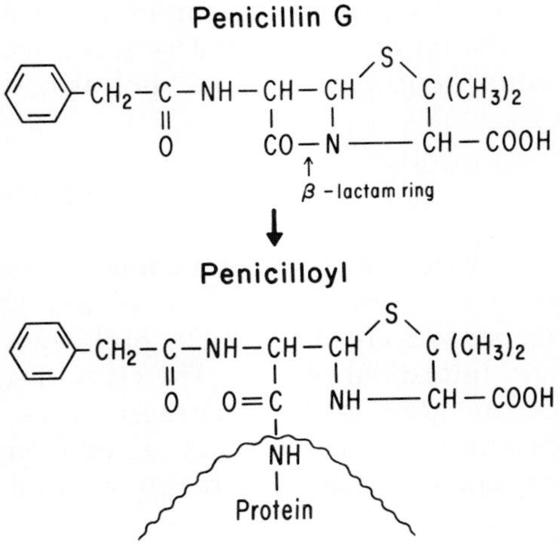

Figure 7–4. Formation of antigenic penicilloyl hapten.

using an alternative antibiotic in patients with a history of penicillin allergenicity. However, sensitization of a patient may occur without their knowledge. For example, drinking milk from a cow treated with penicillin is a common cause. Cross allergenicity exists between penicillins and cephalosporins; these should, therefore, be avoided in patients allergic to penicillin.

Sensitivity to penicillin can be assessed by determining the response to a benzylpenicilloyl-polylysine skin test. Patients with a positive response are at significant risk of developing a serious reaction. Only 3% of patients with negative skin tests have claimed to show allergic reactions to penicillin when treated. In contrast, approximately 75% of patients with positive skin tests show allergic responses. In the event of anaphylaxis, subcutaneous epinephrine (0.3 to 0.5 ml of a 1:1000 solution) is the drug of choice because of its α_1, β_1, and β_2 agonistic properties. Stimulation of these receptors helps to increase peripheral resistance, increase heart rate, and produce bronchodilation. Glucocorticoids and antihistamines may occasionally be useful as secondary therapy.

Drug Induced Asthma

In addition to penicillin-induced anaphylaxis, other drugs can also produce various clinically significant allergenic pulmonary disorders. A relatively common form of drug-induced respiratory disease is asthma. In the asthma-prone individual there is an increasing list of potentially antigenic drugs (Table 7–3). Among these, the most common inducer of asthma is aspirin.

Individuals who have a history of asthma attacks, aspirin hypersensitivity, or nasal polyps are the most likely to react to aspirin (Samter's syndrome). One theory is that aspirin-sensitive asthmatics may differ from nonsensitive asthmatics by relying more on endogenous PGEs than circulatory β-adrenergic agonists for the maintenance of airway patency. Inhibition of cyclooxygenase would then "unmask" the effect of endogenous bronchoconstrictors, such as acetylcholine and histamine.

Alveolitis

Widespread granulomatous inflammatory reactions can occur in the lung as a result of type III allergic responses to various antigens. This response is characterized by proliferation of type II cells, capillary damage, and interstitial fibrosis. The class of drugs that has the greatest number of offenders is the anticancer drugs (Table 7–4). These drugs tend to produce varying degrees of epithelial injury and interstitial fibrosis, depending on dose, duration of treatment, and patient-related factors.

Table 7–3. Pharmacologic Agents Capable of Producing Asthma in Sensitive Individuals

Analgesics	*Autonomics*
Aspirin	Methacholine
Pentazocine	MAO inhibitors
	Parasympathomimetics
Antibiotics	Propranolol
Cephaloridine	
Erythromycin	*Diagnostics*
Ethionamide	Bromsulphalein
Griseofulvin	Radiopaque organic iodides
Neomycin	
Penicillin	*Miscellaneous*
Streptomycin	Acetylcysteine
Tetracycline	Iron dextran
	Mercurials
	Sodium dehydrocholate
	Suxamethonium
	Vitamin K

Table 7–4. Drugs Producing Alveolitis in Humans*

Drug	Pathology	Incidence
Anticancer Agents		
Busulfan	Often large, bizarre granular type II cells; pulmonary fibrosis can appear after several years	2–10% overall incidence
Cyclophosphamide	Similar to busulfan	Rare
Chlorambucil	Similar to busulfan; fibrosis may predominate	Rare
Melphalan	Alveolar epithelial damage more likely than fibrosis	Few reports
Semustine	Alveolar damage, with interstitial fibrosis	One case reported
Bleomycin	Alveolar destruction, interstitial edema, fibrosis	3–5%; more frequent in older patients and in those receiving >400-mg total dose
Mitomycin	Similar to busulfan	Approximately 12 cases reported
Methotrexate	Alveolar and interstitial edema; fibrosis may predominate	More than 40 cases reported
Miscellaneous Agents		
Amiodarone	Pleural and interstitial fibrosis	Several reports
Nitrofurantoin	Acute and chronic effects	Several reports
Hexamethonium; mecamylamine; methysergide; pentolinium	Intra-alveolar fibrinous edema	Rare
Naproxen	Pulmonary infiltrates	Rare

*Inflammation of the alveoli accompanied by a vascular inflammation and bronchiolitis. A more chronic form results in severe respiratory compromise with progressive fibrosis of the lungs.

Allergic alveolitis usually resolves when the patient avoids further exposure to the antigen. However, a short course of glucocorticoids may be necessary to control the pathophysiology. Careful assessment of the patient's clinical, radiologic, and functional status is necessary to determine the need and response of therapy. Prednisolone (40 to 60 mg) is often administered daily for several weeks, whereupon the dosage is gradually reduced over a period of 2 or 3 months.

In addition to their anti-inflammatory effects, glucocorticoids may be used in cases of allergen-induced lung parenchymal disease because they can depress the immune response. This is achieved in a number of ways, including depleting the circulation of lymphocytes by redistribution to other body compartments and preventing the recruitment of additional unstimulated lymphocytes. Glucocorticoids can also lower serum complement levels.

Alveolitis has also been produced in relatively large numbers by the drug nitrofurantoin, with is routinely used for the treatment of urinary tract bacterial infections. Studies in Sweden suggest that pneumotoxicity from nitrofurantoin may be more likely than previously thought. Of those patients who developed lung lesions, over 50% required hospitalization.

Amiodarone is a powerful antiarrhythmic that is structurally related to thyroxine. Within the last several years, this drug has been responsible for at least 14 reported cases of pulmonary toxicity. These include hypersensitivity pneumonitis (2 cases), pulmonary fibrosis (11 cases), and acute necrotizing pneumonitis (1 case). Patients presented with such nonspecific signs and symptoms as progressive dyspnea, fatigue, fever, cough, pleuritic pain, dry basilar rales, and decreased total lung capacity. The cumulative dose of amiodarone prior to the diagnosis of pulmonary toxicity ranged from 12 to 226 g but usually exceeded 128 g. Recovery was achieved with steroid treatment.

Although originally thought to be dose-dependent, data obtained from five cases of amiodarone-associated pneumonitis seem to suggest that the condition is immunologically mediated. All five patients developed pulmonary complications on low-dose treatment (100 to 200 mg/day for 7 to 42 months), and were highly responsive to steroids. In addition, bronchoalveolar lavage revealed high levels of lymphocytes, polymorphonuclear leucocytes, eosinophils, and mast cells.

Pulmonary Eosinophilia

A number of drugs can produce an eosinophil-rich pulmonary infiltrate that can progress to pulmonary fibrosis. The list includes nitrofurantoin, aminosalicylic acid, sulphasalazine, imipramine, phenylbutazone, gold, aspirin, and penicillin. The mechanism appears to involve specific IgE antibodies.

REFERENCES

Adkinson, H. F., Schulman, E. S., and Newball, H. H.: Anaphylactic release of arachidonic acid metabolites from the lung. *In* Newball, H. H. (ed.): Lung Biology in Health and Disease, Vol. 19, New York, Marcell Dekker, 1983, pp. 55–69.

Bienenstock, J.: The lung as an immunologic organ. Ann. Rev. Med., 35:49, 1984.

Eiser, N. M., et al.: The role of histamine receptors in asthma. Clin. Sci., 60:363, 1981.

Leech, J. A., Gallastegui, J., and Swiryn, S.: Pulmonary toxicity of amiodarone. Chest, 85:444, 1984.

Lehnert, B., and Schachter, E.: Airway immunology in health and disease. *In*: The Pharmacology of Respiratory Care, St. Louis, C. V. Mosby, 1980, pp. 60–73.

Parker, C. W.: Immunopharmacology of slow-reacting substance of anaphylaxis. *In* Newball, H. H. (ed.): Lung Biology in Health and Disease, Vol. 19, New York, Marcell Dekker, 1983, pp. 25–45.

Piper, P.: Anaphylaxis and the release of active substance in the lungs. *In* Widdicombe, J. G. (ed.): Respiratory Pharmacology, Section 104, International Encyclopedia of Pharmacology and Therapeutics, Oxford, Pergamon Press, 1981, pp. 705–731.

Skidmore, I. F.: Allergic asthma and rhinitis: The relationship between pathobiology and treatment. Trends Pharm. Sci., 3:66, 1982.

Taskinen, E., Tukiainen, P., and Sovijarvi, A. R. A.: Nitrofurantoin-induced alterations in pulmonary tissue. Acta Pathol. Microbiol. Scand. [A], 85:713, 1977.

Mucokinetic Agents, Radionuclides, and Anticoagulant-Thrombolytic Agents

CHAPTER **8**

MUCOKINETIC AGENTS

The effective maintenance of healthy airway mucous flow (clearance) requires healthy cilia, adequate volumes of normal viscosity secretions, and an operating cough mechanism. However, there are a number of pulmonary diseases, including chronic bronchitis, asthma, pneumonia, and cystic fibrosis, in which one or more of these factors is compromised. In cystic fibrosis, for example, studies indicate decreased permeability of epithelial cells to Cl^- secretion. It has been suggested that this results in a shift in transepithelial liquid flow away from the lumen that concentrates mucus on the airway surface.

Throughout the years, various pharmacologic agents have been employed to assist in the mobilization and evacuation of obstructing secretions that impair ventilation. Unfortunately, lack of interest and poor methods of studying mucociliary activity have contributed to the absence of new drug development, as well as to the accumulation of drugs of questionable efficacy.

The prevailing mucokinetic agents used today can be classified as diluents, surface-active agents, expectorants, or mucolytics. The efficacy of their ingredients is, unfortunately, highly variable and, in some cases, probably nonexistent. The problem is the absence of well-designed double-blind clinical studies. In any event, the mobilization of sputum, if in fact it can be achieved, is usually the result of either hydration (topical, systemic), mucolysis (alteration in molecular bonds), irritation (reflex), or hypertonicity (increased mucosal fluid of low viscosity—bronchorrhea). A summary of mucokinetic agents and probable mechanism(s) of action is shown in Table 8–1.

130

Diluents

As might be expected, the overall state of body hydration appears to have an effect on a secretory apparatus such as the mucociliary escalator. Animal studies, both *in vivo* and *in vitro,* demonstrate that water deprivation results in increased viscocity of airway mucus, with a corresponding decrease in transport velocity. In humans, dehydration in patients with chronic obstructive lung disease is also associated with difficulty in evacuating airway secretions. Presumably, dehydration results in the formation and secretion of a hyperviscous mucus with a depleted sol layer. These effects can be reversed by rehydration.

There is no universal consensus in regard to the most efficient route of water administration. On the one hand, systemic hydration would appear to have the advantage of supplying the water to the site of mucous secretion, production, and transport—the mucosal glands. However, aerosol administration of water is also believed to reduce the viscosity of the gel layer. The process of aerosolization is important, because humidity alone has little effect on mucous viscosity. Aerosolized water administered by ultrasonic nebulization must be used with caution in patients with chronic bronchitis or asthma. These patients have hyperresponsive airways, and are prone to develop reflex bronchospasm. Concurrent administration of β_2-adrenergic amines can protect against this local effect.

Various concentrations of sodium chloride are frequently employed

Table 8–1. Summary of Mucokinetic Agents

Category	Probable Mechanism of Action
Diluent	
Water	Aerosol: Decreases viscosity of gel layer; systemic: increases of sol layer hydration
Saline solution	Hypotonic aerosol: transfer of water from particles to luminal mucus; hypertonic aerosol: osmotic effect of saline, drawing water from the mucosa
Surface-Active	
Propylene glycol	Altered hydration and hydrogen bonding of mucous glycoproteins
Sodium bicarbonate	Decreased mucous viscosity and adhesion, increased ciliary activity
Expectorant	
Potassium iodide	May include stimulation of glands, vagal reflex, or ciliary activity, as well as a direct mucolytic effect or potentiation of proteases
Glyceryl guaiacolate	Vagal stimulation and direct action on bronchial glands
Ammonium chloride	Vagal stimulation and possible enhanced ciliary activity
Mucolytic	
Acetylcysteine	Destruction of disulfide bonds
Dornase	Direct digestion of DNA and indirect enhancement of mucous proteolysis

in aerosol therapy. Nebulization of these solutions can also induce bronchospasm in sensitive individuals. In a study designed to investigate the effect of solution tonicity on airway response, asthmatic subjects with nonspecific airway reactivity received one of four nebulized solutions: commercially available ipratropium bromide in hypotonic saline; hypotonic saline alone; ipratropium bromide in isotonic saline; or isotonic saline alone. The results of this study indicated that, in this group of patients, both hypotonic solutions caused bronchoconstriction, with maximum falls of FEV_1 of 48 to 56 percent. The bronchoconstriction was reversed when the vehicle was adjusted to isotonicity. The effect of hypertonicity was not investigated in this study, but coughing is generally more frequent with hypertonic saline.

Half-normal saline appears to be the most popular diluent when the aerosol is administered by ultrasonic nebulization. It has been claimed that water loss from these hypotonic salt particles results in hydration of luminal mucus and deeper penetration of the particles. Theoretically, hypertonic saline should also be effective by osmotically attracting fluid out of the mucosa, thereby adding water to the respiratory secretions and improving mucokinesis. Inhalation of hypertonic saline has been reported to be effective in the management of cystic fibrosis.

Surface-Active Agents

Surface-active agents are believed to decrease the adhesiveness of airway secretions to the intraluminal walls, but they have no mucolytic activity. The two main examples of this group are propylene glycol and sodium bicarbonate.

Propylene glycol, being hygroscopic, absorbs moisture and is freely soluble in water. It has been suggested that propylene glycol disorganizes mucus by altering its level of hydration and by disrupting cross linking hydrogen bonds. The use of propylene glycol is associated with the stabilization of aerosol droplets, and with a narrow spectrum of disinfectant activity. Propylene glycol has been used alone or in combination with hypertonic saline to induce coughing for the production of a sputum sample. In high doses, propylene glycol can irritate the upper airway and lungs. Concentrations of up to 80% do not appear to produce serious toxicity, however.

There is some evidence to indicate that mucus becomes less adhesive and more susceptible to natural proteases in an alkaline environment. Hence, sodium bicarbonate administered by aerosol has been used. An additional mucokinetic effect suggested for sodium bicarbonate is an increase of ciliary activity. Because sodium bicarbonate is usually administered in concentrations ranging from 2 to 7.5%, these solutions are hypertonic, which may be significant because hypertonicity itself may result in a direct mucolytic effect. As was the case with saline and propylene glycol, high concentrations of sodium bicarbonate can be irritating, and produce bronchospasm and coughing. Sodium bicarbonate has also been recommended as a diluent for acetylcysteine (see below) and as a vehicle for bronchodilators.

Expectorants

Agents in this category include ammonium chloride, potassium iodide, and glyceryl guaiacolate. These drugs have been used in an attempt to improve clearance of secretions in those with chronic obstructive pulmonary disease. Although many patients and clinicians are convinced of their usefulness, there is little human data to substantiate such convictions. Animal studies do indicate that these agents can increase the volume of secretions, with possible reduced viscosity. However, large doses had to be used.

Potassium iodide has been a popular expectorant and is usually administered orally, either in solution or as enteric-coated tablets, although intravenous drip can be used if necessary. Toxic side effects are those associated with iodism, and include skin rash, parotitis, lacrimal gland enlargement, and fever. Particular care should be exercised with chronic use, because suppression of thyroid gland activity may occur. Iodide should be administered with particular care to pregnant women, because fetal goiter development is possible. It has also been suggested that enteric-coated potassium iodide tablets are associated with nonspecific small bowel lesions. Potassium iodide is preferably used only for short-term treatment; its effectiveness as an expectorant is in doubt.

Glyceryl guaiacolate is a mixture of phenols, consisting mainly of creosol and guaiacol. As mentioned previously, glyceryl guaiacolate is found in various cough medications (see Chap. 6), and has been reported to increase mucociliary clearance in chronic bronchitis. It is administered orally and may produce gastric irritation, with nausea and vomiting. Opinion is widespread on the utility of this agent, and the literature contains numerous conflicting studies. Its effectiveness, at this time, remains highly controversial

Ammonium chloride is found in a number of expectorant mixtures. It has been reported to increase mucosal secretions, although less so than potassium iodide. Its use should be limited in patients with electrolyte disturbances, because sodium retention may occur. Ammonium chloride may produce metabolic acidosis when given in large doses. Its effectiveness is also in doubt.

Mucolytics

In many types of lung disorders there is an overproduction of mucus in the respiratory tract, which contributes to an accumulation of sputum (DNA, and cell debris). This can occur as a result of genetic predisposition (*e.g.*, cystic fibrosis), chronic exposure to a pneumotoxin (*e.g.*, cigarette smoking), asthma, or infections. If the excess sputum is not cleared effectively, it will tend to accumulate in smaller airways (primarily bronchioles), interfere with gas exchange, and serve as a site for infection.

The principal mucolytic drug currently available is the sulfhydryl compound acetylcysteine. Acetylcysteine was introduced in the early 1960s and is the most popular proprietary mucolytic agent. It has been found to be beneficial after aerosol administration in certain cases of viscid mucus (*e.g.*, bronchitis, asthma, emphysema). Other applications include patients with atelectases and those with an indwelling endotracheal tube. Its use in cystic fibrosis is controversial, but may have application in selected cases. Conditions associated with purulent (cell-rich) sputum, such as bronchiectasis and pneumonia, would not appear to be affected as much by acetylcysteine because of the presence of additional high-molecular-weight substances, such as nucleic acids.

Acetylcysteine is usually administered as its sodium salt by inhalation or instillation. When given by nebulizer (via face mask, mouthpiece, or tracheostomy), 1 to 10 ml of a 20% solution or 2 to 20 ml of a 10% solution may be nebulized every 2 to 6 hours. The recommended dose for most patients is 3 to 5 ml of the 20% solution or 6 to 10 ml of the 10% solution three to four times a day. Direct instillation (*e.g.*, tracheostomy) involves 1 to 2 ml of a 10 to 20% solution, given as often as every hour. The drug is most effective when directly instilled into the respiratory tract, and results are much more impressive than those obtained by nebulizing the drug, because a higher concentration is achieved at the site of action. The use of sodium bicarbonate as a diluent may maximize acetylcysteine's effect, because its pH optimum is in the range of 7 to 9. Acetylcysteine is also available with the bronchodilator isoproterenol, but its use should be limited to nebulization or to inhalation using a face mask or mouthpiece (together with a tent).

The mechanism of action of acetylcysteine is dependent on its sulfhydryl group, which is thought to reduce the disulfide bonds that bridge the mucoproteins in mucin (Fig. 8–1). This decrease in intermolecular binding results in a corresponding change in molecular shape and in increased flow characteristics. Disadvantages of acetylcysteine use include an unpleasant odor (from hydrogen sulfide liberation) and possible reflex bronchospasm (particularly in asthmatics with hyperactive airways).

RADIONUCLIDES

Advances in nuclear medicine have made, and are continuing to make, significant contributions for investigation of suspected pulmonary vascular abnormalities. For example, perfusion scanning (*i.e.*, blood flow) studies play a critical role in the diagnosis of pulmonary embolism.

Pulmonary studies employing radionuclides offer the advantages of low risk and cost, with more versatility than angiographic techniques (*i.e.*, vessel patency). It is not surprising, therefore, that lung scanning is replacing angiography in the assessment of pulmonary vascular status.

^{131}I-Labeled Albumin

One of the first radioactive labels used for displaying the pulmonary vasculature was iodine-131 (^{131}I). This radioisotope was combined with macroaggregates of albumin, ranging in size from 5 to 100 μm. Following intravenous administration, the particles become trapped in small pulmonary vessels, in which they persist for 2 to 9 hours before being disaggregated. During the period of entrapment, scanning can be carried out.

The use of ^{131}I-tagged albumin is associated with three major disadvantages, however. For example, in patients with severe pulmonary hypertension or diffuse obliterative pulmonary vascular disease, additional vascular blockage by the macroaggregate can cause acute pulmonary hypertension or even death. In addition, the relatively long half-life of ^{131}I (8 days) requires the administration of low doses to reduce exposure, which can produce lung scans lacking in definition. A final disadvantage of this radiopharmaceutical is accumulation by the thyroid, with possible gland damage.

MUCOPROTEIN CHAIN

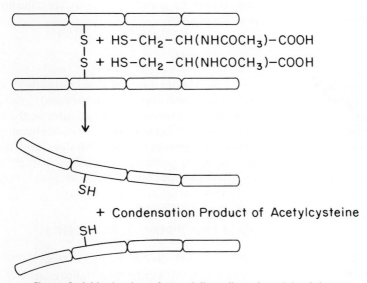

$$S + HS-CH_2-CH(NHCOCH_3)-COOH$$
$$S + HS-CH_2-CH(NHCOCH_3)-COOH$$

SH

+ Condensation Product of Acetylcysteine

SH

Figure 8–1. Mechanism of mucolytic action of acetylcysteine.

^{99m}Tc-Labeled Albumin

Technetium-99m (^{99m}Tc) is a gamma ray emitter artificially produced from molybdenum by a radionuclide generator. It is the most widely used radionuclide for lung scanning, and is available as an albumin macroaggregate or as albumin microsphere particles, with the former being the agent of choice. Advantages over ^{131}I include shorter half-life (6 hours), no thyroid gland accumulation, and safe use of larger doses, producing technically superior lung scans. Iron hydroxide that was formerly used as a carrier of technetium is declining in use because of its adverse effects. Aerosol deposition of ^{99m}Tc has been reported to be sensitive to small airway dysfunction in asthmatic subjects, implying distinct disturbance of interregional ventilation. A relatively new radionuclide, Indium-113m, has been reported to produce excellent lung scans comparable to those of technetium.

^{133}Xe Gas

This short-lived radioactive gas can be used for visualizing the circulation and ventilatory distribution of the lung. When dissolved in physiologic saline and administered intravenously, 90% of xenon-133 (^{133}Xe) is removed by the pulmonary vasculature during its first pass. To obtain an image, the breath is held at total lung capacity for 15 seconds; imaging during breath-holding provides a picture of the circulation. When breathing resumes, ^{133}Xe diffuses throughout the lung, revealing ventilatory distribution. Ventilatory distribution within the lung can also be assessed by inhalation of ^{133}Xe. As the patient breathes a ^{133}Xe air mixture, a series of photoscans are taken to determine both distribution and elimination from the various lung areas.

^{67}Ga

The isotope gallium-67-(^{67}Ga) has been found to accumulate in various lung lesions, including neoplastic (carcinomas, lymphomas), granulomatous (sarcoidosis), and inflammatory lesions. The more intense the inflammatory process, the more intense the ^{67}Ga uptake. ^{67}Ga concentrations can reveal very small carcinomas and pneumonitis infiltrates, and assist in differentiating them from nonseptic pulmonary infarcts, which do not sequester the radioactivity. Because uptake of ^{67}Ga is slow, scans are usually taken 48 hours after intravenous administration.

ANTICOAGULANT AND THROMBOLYTIC AGENTS

Acute pulmonary embolism that obstructs more than 50% of the pulmonary vascular bed causes right ventricular failure and a fall in cardiac output. It has been estimated that pulmonary embolism is the third most common cause of death in the United States (100,000 annually). Symptomatic episodes occur three times more often than strokes.

Most pulmonary emboli originate from venous thrombi formed in calf and thigh veins (*e.g.,* iliofemoral). Three factors are believed to be important in the genesis of thrombi: structural changes in the vessel wall (platelet aggregation); decreased blood flow (stasis plus triggering factor can produce thrombosis); and increased coagulability of the blood (elevated coagulation factors). A number of factors and conditions have been identified that can increase the risk of an individual to venous thromboembolism and, hence, to pulmonary embolism; these include immobilization, increasing age, trauma or burn, pregnancy and parturition, use of oral contraceptives, obesity, varicose veins, previous history of venous thromboembolism, congestive heart failure and atrial fibrillation, and pancreatic, gastric, or pulmonary cancer. It has been estimated that death occurs in 11% of all cases of pulmonary embolism within 1 hour, and 50% of those die within 15 minutes. Additional deaths can occur within several hours as a result of the development of more emboli.

The main goal of anticoagulant therapy is to prevent the development of new thrombi and to allow natural fibrinolysis of pre-existing thrombi to occur. Treatment of pulmonary embolism with antithrombotic drugs can prevent recurrence and reduce mortality. The anticoagulants heparin and coumarins are used for prophylaxis and treatment of venous thrombosis and pulmonary embolism, while thrombolytic agents are employed for the rapid dissolution of obstructing thrombi. However, by their very nature, antithrombotic drugs carry a high risk of untoward bleeding.

Anticoagulants

Blood coagulation is the product of a sequential activation of specific plasma proteins following tissue injury. The result is a deposition of an insoluble fibrin clot. The clotting factors involved are primarily intrinsic to the blood, with the exception of tissue thromboplastin (extrinsic; Fig. 8–2). Antagonism of the clotting pathway can be achieved, therefore, either by reducing the synthesis of the inactive precursors, or by inhibiting the activation of the precursors.

Warfarin. Reducing the synthesis of inactive precursors is exemplified by the coumarin derivative warfarin, which is the prototypic oral anticoagulant.The hepatic synthesis of clotting factors VII, IX, X, and prothrombin requires the availability of fat-soluble vitamin K_1. As can be seen from Figure 8–3, warfarin bears a close structural similarity to vitamin K_1. Coumarin-type drugs interfere with the vitamin K cycle by blocking the enzyme (vitamin K epoxide reductase) that reduces vitamin K_1 epoxide to vitamin K_1. The result is decreased carboxylation of glutamic acid residues of clotting factors VII, IX, X, and prothrombin, thereby inhibiting their activation. In view of the fact that pre-existing clotting factors will be

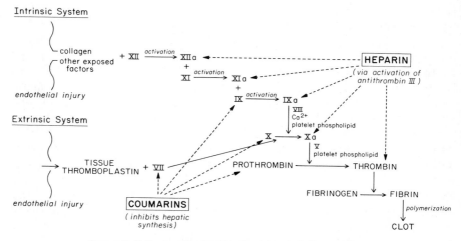

Figure 8–2. Factors involved in the blood clotting pathway.

unaffected, a delay in the anticoagulant effect is inevitable until the normal circulating clotting factors have been metabolized (18 to 72 hours).

Warfarin is well absorbed from the gastrointestinal tract, whereupon it is extensively bound to plasma albumin (99% of the racemic mixture). The albumin-warfarin complex serves as a reservoir, dissociating as the free drug concentration is lowered by distribution and biotransformation (hepatic hydroxylation). The high level of albumin binding is a principal factor in warfarin's prolonged half-life (37 ± 15 hours) and in its slow change in steady state concentration after adjustment to the maintenance dose. The patient's maintenance dose is determined by bioassay—that is, the amount needed to increase the prothrombin time from 2 to 2½ times

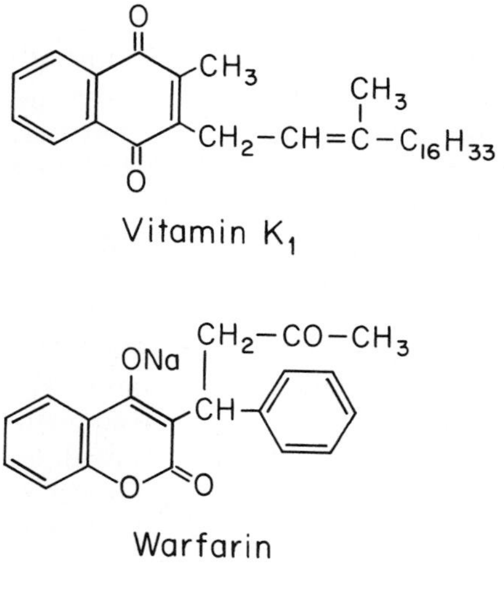

Vitamin K_1

Figure 8–3. Structural comparison of vitamin K_1 and warfarin.

Warfarin

normal (usually 1 to 15 mg). The wide range in maintenance dose is caused by a correspondingly wide variation in human metabolism of warfarin.

The most probable side effect produced by an oral anticoagulant such as warfarin is microscopic bleeding. This can occur spontaneously in cases of overdosage or as an exacerbation of traumatic bleeding when used in the therapeutic range. The specific antidote for oral anticoagulant-induced bleeding is vitamin K_1. It is given intravenously at a rate of 5 mg/minute for a period of 6 to 12 hours to restore the prothrombin time to a safe level. In emergency situations, serious bleeding can be antagonized by stopping the drug and by administering fresh-frozen plasma or factor concentrates containing the necessary coagulation proteins. Oral anticoagulant therapy is contraindicated in cases of malignant hypertension, recent stroke, active peptic ulceration, bleeding diathesis, gastrointestinal bleeding, alcoholism, and during the first trimester of pregnancy.

A number of drugs are known to interact with oral anticoagulants, which therefore alter their pharmacodynamics and anticoagulant effect. The various interactive mechanisms include the following: (1) an increase or decrease in gastric absorption; (2) displacement from albumin binding sites (*e.g.*, phenylbutazone); (3) increased (*e.g.*, barbiturates) or decreased (*e.g.*, phenylbutazone) hepatic metabolism; (4) reduced vitamin K_1 absorption (*e.g.*, neomycin or tetracycline use in surgery patients); and (5) impaired platelet function (*e.g.*, aspirin). It is important to appreciate that if therapy with a drug affecting the pharmacokinetics of oral anticoagulants is altered, an appropriate adjustment in anticoagulant dosage will have to be made.

Warfarin is routinely used in pulmonary medicine to maintain anticoagulation in acute patients who have suffered a pulmonary embolism. Treatment is carried out until the causative factors have been corrected or, if needed, indefinitely.

The prophylactic use of warfarin is not as clear. Although some evidence exists suggesting a beneficial effect of warfarin in reducing mortality from pulmonary embolism in selected cases (elderly patients with hip fracture), its prophylactic use is not encouraged because of the need for close laboratory control and the risk of bleeding. Dextran 70 or 75 has also been advocated for prophylaxis of venous thromboembolism, but there is insufficient evidence to justify its routine use.

Heparin. As mentioned above, the anticoagulant effect produced by warfarin and by other oral agents is not manifested for many hours following administration. This precludes the use of the oral drugs in cases in which anticoagulation must be produced rapidly. Fortunately, a complex mixture of sulfated mucopolysaccharides found in many animal tissues (*e.g.*, lung and intestinal mucosa) can produce rapid anticoagulation. This material is known as heparin and is commercially prepared from bovine or porcine sources.

As indicated in Figure 8–2, heparin is believed to produce its anticoagulant effect by activating antithrombin III. This is achieved by its binding reversibly to the globulin and inducing a conformational change, which increases its affinity (1000-fold) for thrombin. Subsequent inactivation of thrombin is almost instantaneous because of the formation of a stable complex. The heparin-antithrombin III complex is also believed to inhibit other activated factors.

Heparin must be given parenterally because it is not absorbed from the gastrointestinal tract. Dosage depends on the use intended—that is, whether for established thrombosis or for prophylaxis. In the case of the former, a high dose of heparin is routinely given intramuscularly in a loading dose of 5,000 U followed by a maintenance dose of 30,000 to 40,000 U daily for the first 48 hours and is reduced to 20,000 to 25,000 U thereafter for up to 7 to 10 days. Larger doses should be restricted for patients in shock. The dose of heparin is adjusted to keep the clotting time between 25 and 30 minutes. When heparin is followed by warfarin therapy, the two drugs should be overlapped for 2 to 3 days until the warfarin effect has been established.

If heparin is used prophylactically, it is given subcutaneously in a dose of 5,000 U every 8 or 12 hours (low dose). Its success depends on the neutralization of factor X_a (increased following surgery), which prevents formation of the thrombus. Higher doses of heparin are needed for established thrombosis because a preformed thrombus can catalyze its own production via an aggregating effect on platelets. Heparin is the drug most commonly used to prevent venous thrombosis.

As with the oral anticoagulants, bleeding is the most common side effect, and occurs in 20% of treatment courses. Serious bleeding is believed to occur in approximately 10% of courses. In the case of heparin-induced bleeding, patients should receive 50 mg of protamine sulfate over 10 minutes given by the intravenous route. This basic peptide combines with the acidic heparin and inactivates it. However, the appropriate dose of protamine depends on the dose of heparin: 1 mg of protamine is sufficient to inactivate approximately 100 U of heparin. Only 50% of this dose is required if 1 hour has elapsed since the heparin was administered because of its rapid clearance. In 5 to 10% of patients, heparin may induce thrombocytopenia. Heparin should be discontinued if the platelet count drops below 75,000/µl. Therefore, the platelet count should be measured twice weekly. Chronic heparin treatment (6 months) may result in osteoporosis and alopecia.

Fibrinolytic Drugs

Two fibrinolytic drugs are available that have been used successfully in the treatment of massive pulmonary embolism. These are the enzymes streptokinase and urokinase. Streptokinase is normally synthesized by group C β-hemolytic streptococci, while urokinase is produced commercially from cultured human fetal kidney cells. Experts have determined that these two enzymes are the agents of choice for treating pulmonary embolism in selected cases.

These drugs differ from heparin and warfarin in that they act to break down clots already formed rather than to inhibit clot formation. They are effective for only 5 to 7 days after embolism has occurred. Their mechanism of action involves the generation of a protease (plasmin) within the thrombus that catalyzes the breakdown of the fibrin aggregate (Fig. 8–4). In the case of streptokinase, it combines with plasminogen in a 1:1 complex to produce a conformational activation. The enzyme is reconstituted by sequential fragmentation of the streptokinase. Urokinase, on the other hand, is a direct activator of plasminogen.

Both drugs are administered intravenously on a fixed-dose schedule. A loading dose of streptokinase (250,000 U) is given over 30 minutes to saturate circulating levels of the antistreptococcal antibodies that are usually present. This overcomes the neutralization effect of the antibodies and allows excess enzyme to combine with plasminogen. The streptokinase maintenance dose is 100,000 U/hour for 24 hours in cases of pulmonary embolism, using a constant rate infusion pump. After treatment has been discontinued, heparin is administered and, if warranted, an oral anticoagulant may be substituted later. The cost of this product is not insignificant; in 1982, a standard course of streptokinase cost approximately 275 dollars. Allergic reactions occur in 5 to 10% of patients receiving streptokinase.

The loading dose of urokinase is 4400 U/kg body weight infused over 10 minutes, followed by continuous administration of 4400 U/kg/hour for 12 to 24 hours in cases of pulmonary embolism. After thrombolytic therapy has been completed, systemic heparin should be continued for 5 to 10

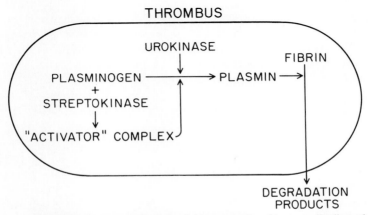

Figure 8–4. Comparison of streptokinase and urokinase activation of thrombus plasminogen.

days, followed by oral anticoagulants (if needed). Urokinase has a short half-life (15 minutes) and is nonantigenic in humans, but its cost is about tenfold that of streptokinase. If excessive bleeding is induced during fibrinolytic therapy, the drug should be stopped and fibrinogen administered, either as fresh-frozen plasma or as fibrinogen concentrates.

With the advent of genetic engineering, many of the more clinically important human proteins are being produced. For example, tissue plasminogen activator is known to be a more specific and potent fibrinolytic agent than urokinase. Unfortunately, only small amounts can be isolated, but it has recently been reported that tissue plasminogen activator has been successfully expressed in *Escherichia coli*. The production of tissue plasminogen activator on a large scale will make possible its clinical trial as a thrombolytic agent in humans.

SELECTED REFERENCES

Luderer, J. R.: Anticoagulant, thrombolytic, and antiplatelet drugs. *In* Goth, A.. (ed.): Modern Pharmacology, St. Louis, C. V. Mosby, 1984, pp. 460–470.
Richardson, P. S., and Phipps, R. J.:. The anatomy, physiology, pharmacology and pathology of tracheobronchial mucus secretion and the use of expectorant drugs in human disease. *In* Widdicombe, J. G. (ed.): Respiratory Pharmacology, Section 104, International Encyclopedia of Pharmacology and Therapeutics, Oxford, Pergamon Press, 1981, pp. 437–475.
Sherry, S., Bell, W. R., Duckert, F. H., Fletcher, A. P., Gurewich, V., Long, D. M., Marder, V. J., Roberts, H. R., Salzman, E. W., Sasahara, A., and Verstraete, M.: Thrombolytic therapy in thrombosis: A National Institute of Health Development Conference. Ann. Intern. Med., 93:141, 1980.
Wall, R. T.: Drugs used in disorders of coagulation. *In* Katzung, B. G. (ed.): Basic and Clinical Pharmacology, Los Altos, Lange Medical Publications, 1982, pp. 345–353.
Ziment, I.: Mucokinetic agents. *In* Ziment, I.: Respiratory Pharmacology and Therapeutics, Philadelphia, W. B. Saunders, 1978, pp. 60–104.

CHAPTER 9

Responses of the Lung to Injury

DEFENSE MECHANISMS

Because the respiratory system provides a portal through which noxious agents may gain access to the body, it became necessary for our species to develop a number of defense mechanisms. Some of these mechanisms are unique to the respiratory system, and are relatively complex because they tend to be specifically modified for the various regions of the respiratory system.

The following are examples of the major physiologic defense mechanisms that may be elicited in the respiratory system in response to inhaled material: *reflex* mechanisms include sneezing, swallowing, coughing, and apnea; *removal* processes include mucociliary transport and actions of the lymphatic system and of macrophages; and *cellular* processes include morphometric, inflammatory, and fibrotic reactions. Those factors that will be operative at a given time are dependent on the relevant physical and chemical characteristics of the material in question. It should be kept in mind, however, that not all these mechanisms are exclusively restricted to inspired material, but can also be invoked against bloodborne toxicants.

The most rapid responses that the body can have to inhaled materials are those aimed at stopping and removing the invading material from the respiratory pathway. Reflexes have the advantage of being fast responses in situations in which delay could be fatal. If this rapid defense system fails, then an intruding material may be removed more slowly over a period of hours or days by mucociliary transport, macrophage ingestion, or local removal by lymphatics. If the offending material achieves sufficient contact with tissue there can be local cellular reactions to injury, including cellular proliferation, inflammation, and fibrosis. In practice, these patterns of response are rarely isolated but usually occur sequentially or simultaneously.

Reflexes

Exposure of the upper airway to irritant gases such as sulfur dioxide stimulates sensory fibers in irritant receptors located in the larynx and bronchi. Activation of these fibers causes a reflex constriction of the lower airway (bronchioles) to block subsequent passage of the gas. A similar effect can be caused by exposure to ammonia, ozone, sulfuric acid, or phosgene. Stimulation of irritant receptors in the tracheal epithelium can also cause coughing in an attempt to expel the material.

Receptors in the larynx, trachea, and bronchi can also be stimulated by dust particles (*e.g.*, cigarette smoke, carbon dust), and can cause significant reflex bronchoconstriction. Insoluble dusts are believed to act as mechanical stimuli. This reflex bronchoconstriction can be abolished by vagotomy or by the administration of acetylcholine-blocking drugs, indicating parasympathetic involvement. The bronchoconstriction produced by the inhalation of dust particles will tend to last longer than that produced by irritant gases, because particles must be cleared by the slow mucociliary pathway.

As noted in Chapter 1, there is a group of afferent sensory fibers in the distal section of the airway known as J receptors. These fibers differ from those in the upper airway in that their reflex involves a reduction in breathing rather than bronchoconstriction. Activation of J receptors, therefore, produces reflex apnea followed by rapid shallow breathing, as well as hypotension and bradycardia. Both irritant and J receptors respond primarily to nociceptive agents, and travel in the vagi.

Inhalational Provocation Agents

In certain diagnostic circumstances, potential toxins are intentionally given by inhalation to elicit bronchospasm. The response of the individual patient is then monitored using a physiologic parameter such as the amount of air that can be expelled in 1 second (forced expiratory volume, or FEV_1). This type of provocative exposure can be used to identify an offending material, determine the patient's sensitivity to it, and assess the magnitude of the response.

Over the years, a large number of irritant agents (*e.g.*, drugs, allergens, industrial agents) have been used in pulmonary function laboratories as provocateurs to assist in the diagnosis of asthma. Asthmatics are particularly sensitive to inhaled irritants. Because of the need for special facilities, as well as the potential danger, only adequately prepared laboratories are encouraged to undertake provocation studies.

The most popular drug used in provocation testing is probably methacholine, which is used to determine nonspecific bronchial reactivity. Methacholine is a derivative of acetylcholine, but with more resistance to hydrolysis and with 10 to 20 times the muscarinic potency. Introduced for this purpose in 1947, inhalational administration of methacholine produces bronchoconstriction and bronchial secretion. It is usually administered as an aerosolized solution in graded concentrations using various protocols. The degree of sensitivity to inhaled methacholine correlates with the severity of the asthma. It is important that medication be withheld for a sufficient period of time prior to the test—for example, 8 hours for bronchodilators (12 hours if sustained release), 24 hours for cromolyn, 48 hours for antihistamines, and 96 hours for hydroxyzine.

An alternative to methacholine is histamine. It is marketed as a histamine phosphate solution, and is aerosolized in concentrations ranging from 0.02 to 10 mg/ml. Sequential exposures involve a doubling of the dose. Methacholine and histamine produce bronchoconstriction over the same range of concentrations, and results with the two agents in the same group of asthmatics are very similar. One advantage of histamine is that there is no cumulative effect when administered repeatedly, thereby allowing more precise expression of threshold dose. Although methacholine has a mild cumulative effect, it is, however, better tolerated at high doses than is histamine. In one study, for example, 7 of 47 patients were unable to take the highest concentration of histamine because of adverse effects.

Tracheobronchial Mucus

The importance of the mucous lining of the respiratory tract has been briefly noted in previous chapters. We will now discuss this important protective component in more detail. Tracheobronchial mucus itself is produced by submucosal glands and surface epithelial goblet cells, both of which are numerous in the upper airways but diminish in number in peripheral airways. Studies in the guinea pig indicate that the mucous layer is continuous, extending from the larynx to the end of the first-generation bronchi. Human, submucosal glands occupy approximately 40 times more volume than surface goblet cells and are, therefore, the major contributor to mucous secretion. Clara cells and alveolar type II cells also contribute to airway secretions, but the extent of their contribution is unclear. One theory is that airway irritation induces a transition of Clara cells to goblet cells. Secretion by submucosal glands is under parasympathetic control via the vagus, while the goblet cells appear to respond independently. Estimates of the amount of daily secretion of mucus by the tracheobronchial tree range from 10 to 100 ml.

The chemical composition of mucus is primarily water (roughly 95%). Therefore, in situations in which the water content of mucus is reduced, a more viscous material is produced. This can occur in certain disease states (*e.g.*, cystic fibrosis) and following exposure to certain pneumotoxins. In addition to water, isotonic levels of sodium, calcium, and chloride ions and, most importantly, high-molecular-weight (several million daltons), sugar-rich glycoproteins are found.

Tracheobronchial mucous glycoproteins (mucins) are characterized by the presence of fucose, galactose (sulfated or free), N-acetylgalactosamine, and N-acetylglucosamine in the oligosaccharide (two to ten monosaccharides) side chains along the protein backbone. If present, sialic acid can be found at the nonreducing ends of the oligosaccharides. Protein subunits are cross linked via disulfide bridges between cysteine residues on adjacent protein chains. This cross linking, together with the high frequency of liposaccharide side chains, confers an extremely viscous nature to this material. The component glycoproteins are classified as neutral or acidic (sulfomucins and sialomucins) on the basis of their separation by ion exchange chromatography or by electrophoresis. Irritation of the mucosal membrane by tobacco smoke results in a switch from neutral to acidic glycoproteins.

The molecular weight (MW) of mucin can vary. For example, mucin from cystic fibrosis patients has a higher MW than mucin from asthmatic patients (11.3×10^6 daltons versus 7.2×10^6 daltons). This suggests that mucin exists in varying states of aggregation, which may influence its viscoelastic properties. Mucus that is either too thick or too thin (*e.g.*, as in bronchorrhea) will not be handled efficiently by the cilia.

Bronchial secretions also contain an 11,000 MW protein known as bronchial mucous inhibitor (BMI). The physiologic function of this protein seems to be the control of leukocyte proteases such as elastase and cathepsin G. *In vitro* studies have shown that ozone can abolish BMI's inhibitory activity against proteases, indicating that exposure to high levels of oxidants could compromise the control of leukocyte proteinases by BMI.

Cilia

The current view of the relationship of cilia to the structure of tracheobronchial mucus involves a two-layer model (Fig. 9–1). This stratification arrangement allows most ciliary movement to occur in the less viscous sol layer, thereby conserving energy. When the forward effective stroke achieves its maximum velocity, the tips of the cilia contact the gel layer and move it along. The recovery stroke is slower, taking three times as long as the forward stroke, and occurs in the sol layer. It is not known whether the mucous layer is continuous or discontinuous along the epithelial surface, although present opinion favors the latter.

The cilia in the tracheobronchial area consist of a shaft, a basal body, and a root as the three main structural components. Ultrastructural studies of human cilia reveal a pattern of two central longitudinal fibrils connected to nine pairs of peripheral fibrils by radial spokes (Fig. 9–2). Although not

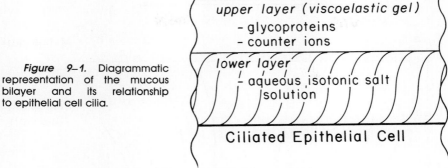

Figure 9–1. Diagrammatic representation of the mucous bilayer and its relationship to epithelial cell cilia.

under neurologic control, they do beat in a coordinated fashion toward the larynx with a metachronous wave pattern, in which parallel ranks of cilia beat one after another and not synchronously (Fig. 9–3). They are believed to beat as a consequence of changes in the lateral bonding of two microtubule filaments, tubulin and dynein. Dynein, which has ATPase activity, is believed to bind and hydrolyze ATP, which produces cyclic changes in shape.

Studies in the rat indicate that, at the tracheal level, there are about 200 cilia/cell, with dimensions of approximately 0.25×5.0 μm. An important feature of mucociliary transport is that cilia beat at successively lower frequencies as airway diameter decreases, resulting in a corresponding decline in mucous velocity (Table 9–1). It is also known that there is considerable variation among individuals in their clearance rates: some people clear particles rapidly from their ciliary airways, while others do

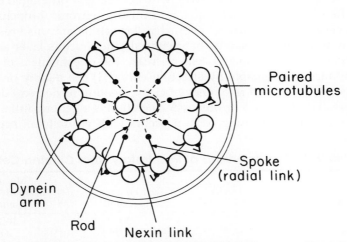

Figure 9–2. Diagrammatic representation of the cross section of a human cilium.

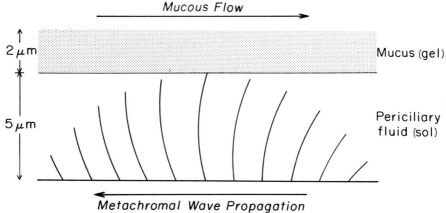

Figure 9–3. Relationship of cilia wave propagation to mucous flow.

this relatively slowly. The normal variation in clearance rate appears to be determined by heredity.

One functional decrement of asthmatic patients is a failure of mucociliary clearance. Studies of the movement of radiopaque particles in the trachea of asthmatics in remission have shown a rate only 50% that of normal. Subsequent antigen challenge slows the rate even further, to only 25% of that found in control subjects. The reduction in mucociliary clearance in asthmatics is believed to be caused by SRS-A, which both increases mucous secretory rate and decreases mucociliary transport.

Some patients (1:20,000) suffer from an "immobilecilia syndrome," which is caused by an autosomal recessive disease producing a deficiency of dynein arms in cilia. This leads to impairment of mucociliary transport in both the upper and lower airways, with consequent prolonged exposure of an offending agent that leads to sinusitis, chronic bronchitis, and bronchiectasis. Severe chronic obstructive bronchitis may also result.

Invariably, pneumotoxins that penetrate the mucous layer and reach mucus-producing and ciliated cells decrease the effectiveness of mucociliary clearance, presumably by affecting either (1) the quality or quantity of mucus (via decreased frequency of ciliary beating or decreased concentration of cilia). Because mucous hypersecretion is a general inflammatory response in mucus-secreting cells, it occurs with virtually all agents that

Table 9–1. Characteristics of Respiratory Tract Ciliated Cells*

Region	Total Cells (%)	Beat Frequency (per min)	Mucous Transport Velocity (mm/min)
Trachea	17	1000	10.1
Bronchioles	65	400	0.6

*These values are approximations, and vary according to source.

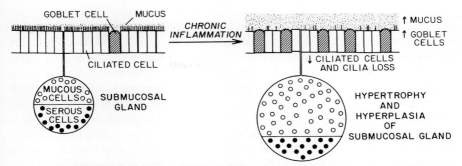

Figure 9–4. Diagram of the effect of chronic inflammation on epithelial cells, mucous, and submucosal glands.

damage the tracheobronchial region. Recent evidence indicates that leukotriene C_4 may be an important mediator of hypersecretion. Under certain conditions, chronic exposure to pulmonary irritants such as cigarette smoke and sulfur dioxide can also lead to a compensatory increase in the number of mucus-secreting cells and to a decrease in ciliated cells (Fig. 9–4). Substance P, which is present in sensory fibers innervating the airway mucosa, is the most potent agonist of canine airway glycoprotein secretion described to date, and may be important as a mediator of irritant-induced mucous hypersecretion in the airway.

The combination of increased mucus and decreased ciliated cells, therefore, serves as a twofold cause of reduced clearance in chronic bronchial injury. A representative listing of several pneumotoxins and their effects on mucociliary clearance is shown in Table 9–2. It seems probable that a given pneumotoxin affects mucous clearance in more than one way. Toxin-impaired ciliary function may, therefore, be an important contributor to the pathogenesis of some obstructive lung diseases. Current research suggests that mucociliary clearance slows down during sleep, indicating that the last cigarette of the day may be the most dangerous. The depression of tracheobronchial clearance by chronic cigarette smoking is reversible, and takes approximately 3 months to return to normal after cessation of smoking.

In addition to toxins, pharmacologic agents also affect mucociliary clearance. Ciliary movement and mucous transport are increased by

Table 9–2. Effects of Various Pneumotoxins on Mucociliary Clearance

Increases Mucous Viscosity	Decreases Number of Cilia Cells	Decreases Cilia Beat Frequency
SO_2	NO_2	Cigarette smoke
H_2SO_4 aerosol	SO_2	
NH_3 vapor	Acrolein	
Ozone		
Chromate		

catecholamines (β-receptor stimulants), methylxanthines, acetylcholine, nicotine, and prostaglandin E_1, and depressed by β-receptor blockers, muscarinic blockers, and promazine. Both increases and decreases in mucociliary activity have been reported for serotonin and histamine. The exact mechanism by which β-adrenergic agonists stimulate mucociliary transport is unclear, but seems to involve ciliary stimulation. The spectrum of drugs that can affect ciliary function is apparently quite wide, because even the ubiquitous aspirin has been reported to produce a small but statistically significant decrease in mucociliary clearance and in transport rate in human studies. Also, the mucous layer itself can dissolve some substances, allowing them to become absorbed into the system.

Macrophages

Insoluble material that reaches the lower alveolar region could be a problem because, in humans, there are no ciliated epithelial cells in this area, and hence no clearance by this mechanism. Fortunately, alveolar clearance of particles can be achieved by macrophages. Macrophages can phagocytize particles as great as 1 μm or more in diameter, and transport them either up into the tracheobronchial region for elimination via the mucociliary escalator or into the lymphatic system, which transports material ino the tracheobronchial lymph nodes (Fig. 9–5). The latter mechanism is substantially slower, and may require several months.

Both organic and inorganic particles that reach the respiratory surface are rapidly ingested by alveolar macrophages. With certain substances (*e.g.*, silica) the ensuring phagocytosis results in the release of lysosomal enzymes, which not only degrade the foreign material but may also injure adjacent lung tissue. Other substances can cause enzyme release with no attendant injury (*e.g.*, starch granules) or with no enzyme release at all (*e.g.*, calcium pyrophosphate salt crystals).

Within limits, macrophage response to foreign material is proportionate to the lung burden imposed. However, brief exposure to very high concentrations (*e.g.*, 300 mg/mm^3 of coal dust) can delay clearance. In addition, prolonged exposure to massive concentrations can cause permanent failure of this mechanism, with resultant accumulation of material and pathologic sequelae.

As mentioned previously, some material deposited in the respiratory system will undergo biotransformation by enzymes located in certain lung cells. However, the body also appears to have less sophisticated mechanisms for dealing with material that might reach the lung. For example, evidence suggests that ammonia (NH_3), normally present in the oral cavity and in nasal passages, can neutralize inhaled sulfuric acid (H_2SO_4) aerosols by forming ammonium bisulfate (NH_4HSO_4) and ammonium sulfate ((NH_4)$_2SO_4$). It has been estimated that, in humans, approximately 1 to

10% neutralization of H_2SO_4 (0.5 μm inhaled at 50% relative humidity) may occur with nose breathing. This is based on a reported NH_3 concentration of 13 to 46 μg/m³ in the human nasal passages.

The suggestion has been made that the extent of H_2SO_4 pollution injury might be somewhat higher in individuals with lower levels of oral cavity ammonia. Because the chief source of oral cavity NH_3 is microorganisms associated with teeth, certain groups of individuals, such as newborns and the elderly, would appear to be in this category. Although the impact of dentition on lung pathology is undoubtedly miniscule, it illustrates the various factors that can interact with inhaled material.

If material that has become deposited in the lung dissolves, it will tend to become evenly distributed by the process of mass action. During this

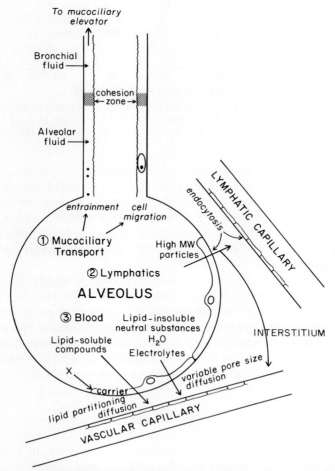

Figure 9–5. Examples of possible routes for clearance of material that has reached the alveoli.

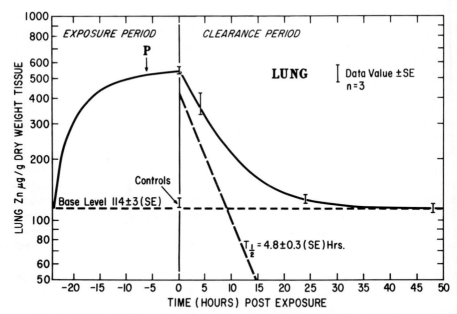

Figure 9–6. Rapid clearance of zinc from the lungs by dissolution and by vascular clearance following exposure of rats to zinc oxide. (From Hollinger, M. A., et al.: Effect of the inhalation of zinc and dietary zinc on paraquat toxicity in the rat. Toxicol. Appl. Pharmacol. 49:58, 1979.)

equilibration, material reaches the capillaries and will be removed from the lung. In the experiment shown in Figure 9–6, small particles of zinc oxide (0.7 to 0.95 μm) were administered to rats by aerosol. After exposure the lungs showed a rapid decline in zinc concentration, which can only be produced by dissolution and vascular clearance. If particles are small enough (less than 0.01 μm), they can pass directly through pores in the alveolar-capillary unit.

In general, the lung has a rather remarkable ability to deal with inhaled dust. The normal bronchial tree, for example, is clean and glistening in appearance despite constant exposure to particle-laden air. Autopsies of elderly city dwellers may reveal gray alveolar tissue, but the total mass of dust in these subjects is only about a few grams. Coal miners who may inhale as much as 5 kg over a lifetime of exposure usually have no more than 40 g of total dust at postmortem examination.

MORPHOMETRY

Most lung diseases caused by chemicals are chronic in nature, such as fibrosis, granuloma formation, emphysema, and cancer. Acute forms of chemically induced lung disease would include pulmonary edema and other types of inflammatory responses. Most current information on the response of the lung to injury is based on the application of electron microscopy, autoradiography, freeze fracture, and modern biochemical techniques. This section will describe cellular changes to injury as well as tissue response and the repair process of selected areas.

Alveolar Region

In general, the alveolar region of the lung shows a stereotypic pattern of response to chemical injury. This tends to be true whether the offending toxicant is introduced through the airways or the bloodstream. Primary morphologic changes include death of type I alveolar epithelial cells and of capillary endothelium. Clara cells, type II cells, and alveolar macrophages appear to be relatively more resistant to injury, which can probably be attributed to their more elaborate complement of defensive intracellular chemical mechanisms.

Injury to epithelial type I cells, for example, can follow inhalation of gases such as ozone, nitrogen dioxide, or high levels of oxygen itself. The exact location and extent of pulmonary damage depends on the particular gas and on its concentration gradient. Ozone and nitrogen dioxide tend to affect terminal bronchioles and adjacent alveoli, while oxygen can affect all regions of the alveoli, including epithelial and endothelial cells.

The systemic administration of agents such as paraquat, bleomycin, butylated hydroxytoluene, nickel carbonyl, thiourea, or 4-ipomeanol tend to produce diffuse damage to the alveoli similar to that reported for oxygen. The extent of damage can vary up to and including complete denudation of the basement membrane. Capillary endothelial cells, although more resistant than type I cells, can also be injured by oxygen, ozone, nitrogen dioxide, nickel carbonyl, pyrrolizidine alkaloids, iprindole, thiourea, and bromocarbamide.

Repair Phase

The response of the lung to injury usually occurs within 24 hours, although the repair process may be delayed in older animals. If type I cells have been damaged, type II cells begin to proliferate. The extent of type II cell proliferation is in direct proportion to the extent of type I cell injury, because the alveolar epithelium is under negative feedback control dependent on the number of differentiated cells present (type I).

Following division, type II cells undergo transformation to type I cells and recover the basement membrane, which takes about 2 days. If the injury has occurred on an acute basis, then the type I cells will develop into normal squamous epithelium. However, under conditions of chronic insult, an intermediate cuboidal epithelium will persist. The presence of this cell type has been associated with the development of tolerance to certain pneumotoxins, although the exact mechanism is unknown.

The increase in cell division that occurs following cellular injury is of course, preceded by increases in nucleic acid levels and in rates of protein synthesis. These anabolic processes have been used as indices of the repair phase in experimental animal models of lung injury.

Other important changes can also occur. For example, an increase in the activity of glucose-6-phosphate dehydrogenase is a common adaptive biochemical response. This undoubtedly reflects an activation of the hexose monophosphate shunt pathway, enabling the lung to increase the production of NADPH for detoxication mechanisms and of pentose for nucleic acid synthesis. Additional enzyme systems, such as selenium-glutathione peroxidase, superoxide dismutase, and ornithine decarboxylase, as well as polyamine content, undoubtedly also play a similarly important role.

Lung hyaluronidase is believed to be significant in affecting the differentiation of proliferated cells. Following hyperoxia-induced lung damage, for example, there is a significant increase in hyaluronidase activity that coincides with that of maximum cell proliferation. It has been suggested that this increase in enzyme activity results in the degradation of a hyaluronate-rich matrix that promotes cell proliferation, and in an increase in sulfate glycosaminoglycans, which favor differentiation of proliferated cells.

Bronchiolar Epithelium

The bronchiolar epithelium is lined with cells that are a continuation of those from the alveoli but that differ morphologically. As mentioned previously, these cells can be divided into ciliated and nonciliated (Clara, intermediate, serous, and brush) cells. Ciliated cells appear to be the most susceptible to injury. Because these cells are involved in the mucociliary escalator, this process can be expected to be compromised early following bronchiolar epithelial damage. Studies on the mechanism for renewal of the bronchiolar epithelium indicate that the Clara cell serves as the progenitor. Like its analog in the alveolar region, the type II cell, it is more resistant to chemical insult (compared to ciliated cells) because of its smaller surface area and its more robust metabolism.

Macrophages

Exposure to environmental (cigarette smoke), occupational (air pollution), or medical (therapeutic oxygen) factors can produce increased susceptibility to respiratory infection, which may partly be attributed to decreased alveolar macrophage function. Exposure of mice to 100% oxygen for 48 and 72 hours, for example, results in reduced bactericidal ability of alveolar macrophages, as measured by uptake of radioactive bacteria. Impaired phagocytosis is the likely cause, because direct exposure of mice alveolar macrophages to 100% oxygen *in vitro* has been demonstrated to reduce their phagocytic potential.

Relatively brief (1 to 7 days) exposure to clinically relevant oxygen tensions appears to impair pulmonary host defense in general, and alveolar macrophage phagocytic function in particular. Exposure of mice and rabbits to other oxidant air pollutants, such as ozone and nitrogen dioxide, has also been reported to depress the ability of alveolar macrophages to phagocytize. In addition, exposure to general anesthetics and trace metal fumes has been reported to inhibit phagocytosis.

The effect of cigarette smoke on alveolar macrophages has also been studied quite extensively. One early demonstrable effect of tobacco smoke is a significant elevation in the macrophage population of the alveoli and of the small bronchioles. Pulmonary lavage of human volunteers indicates a two- to three-fold increase. In addition, macrophages from smokers' lungs tend to be larger, with distinctive brown pigmentation and cytoplasmic inclusions. Furthermore, they are more metabolically active and contain more degradative lysosomal enzymes (*e.g.*, β-glucuronidase, elastase, and lysozyme). Interestingly, however, despite these apparent quantitative advantages, macrophages from smokers' lungs are at best only comparable to nonsmoker macrophages, and in certain cases their performance is inferior. This may partially explain why heavy chronic smoking increases the frequency and severity of lower respiratory tract infections.

Endothelial Cells

The most numerous cells in the lung are pulmonary endothelial cells, and they can also be injured by either airway or bloodborne factors. Their renewal, however, is considerably more straightforward than that of epithelial cells, because no progenitor cells are involved. Instead, endothelial cells are replaced by simple division of pre-existing endothelial cells.

INFLAMMATION

Inflammation is a complex tissue response to injury, and includes such elements as vasodilation and increased vessel permeability, extravasation of serum components, fluid, and cells from blood vessels, the local accumulation of cellular elements, and, finally, healing and repair. The inflammatory process in the lung is augmented by chemical mediators such as histamine, heparin, serotonin, catecholamines, leukotrienes, prostaglandins, and products of the complement, clotting, and kinin systems, as well as by lymphokines.

Mediators

Mediator release in the lung can result in acute (*e.g.*, anaphylaxis) or chronic (*e.g.*, asthma) disability. The ability of the lung to synthesize and release various biologically active substances, therefore, plays an important role in the regulation of pulmonary function and in the mediation of pulmonary injury. Virtually all the current information about this area has been derived from studies of experimental animals. Although confirmation of this data would be desirable in human studies, there are undoubtedly sufficient similarities to render the animal data quite useful. Over a dozen proven and suspected mediators have been identified for the lung. Table 9–3 lists some of those that now appear to play a major role. As can be seen, the mediators are chemically diverse: amines, peptides, proteins, and lipids.

Table 9–3. Miscellaneous Effects Caused by Known or Suspected Mediators Within the Lungs*

Mediator (Source)	Effects
Angiotensin II	Pulmonary vasoconstriction; release of pulmonary prostaglandins; possible role in hypoxic vasoconstriction
Bradykinin (mast cells, basophils)	Pulmonary vasodilation or constriction; bronchoconstriction either directly or via prostaglandin release; release of histamine from mast cells; increase in permeability of pulmonary endothelium
Complement C5a factor	Major mediator of immunologic injury; activation of leukocytes and contraction of smooth muscle
Eosinophil chemotactic factor of anaphylaxis (mast cells, neutrophils, basophils)	Mediates attraction of eosinophils to site of anaphylactic reaction
Histamine (mast cells, basophils)	Possible role in the local regulation of pulmonary blood flow and in hypoxic vasoconstriction; increase in vascular permeability; usually bronchoconstriction; release of arachidonic acid metabolites from lung; increased mucus gland secretion

Table 9–3. Miscellaneous Effects Caused by Known or Suspected
Mediators Within the Lungs* *(Continued)*

Mediator (Source)	Effects
Lymphokines (T-lymphocytes)	Involvement in "cell-mediated" (delayed) hypersensitivity and antibody formation by B-cells for type I reactions
Neurotensin	Degranulation of mast cells and release of histamine
Neutrophil chemotactic factor (mast cells)	Attracts neutrophils
Platelet activating factor (mast cells, neutrophils)	Aggregation and degranulation of platelets; release of serotonin from platelets; does not appear to be a mediator of the allergic reaction in the human nose
Serotonin (mast cells)	Bronchoconstriction; increases synthesis of prostaglandins and platelet aggregation; not a primary mediator in humans
Spasmogenic lung peptide	Constriction of bronchial and vascular smooth muscle
Substance P	Contraction of smooth muscle; stimulates release of mucus and histamine
Vasoactive intestinal peptide	Bronchodilation; protection against bronchoconstriction and vasoconstriction produced by prostaglandins and leukotrienes; inhibition of bronchial mucus production

*Effects vary with species and conditions.

Table 9–4. Some Pulmonary Conditions Associated with Mediator Release

Condition	Mediators
Anaphylaxis	Histamine, ECF-A, bradykinin, leukotrienes, prostaglandins, thromboxane A_2, neutrophil chemotactic factors
Hyperinflation	Prostaglandins, prostacyclin
Hyperventilation	Prostaglandins, prostacyclin
Pulmonary thromboembolism	Histamine, serotonin, prostaglandins
Pulmonary edema	Prostaglandins and thromboxanes
Endotoxin shock	Prostaglandins

Because these mediators are so pharmacologically active, they either are acutely synthesized *de novo* from inactive precursors, or are released from inactive granule stores. In the case of prostaglandins, for example, synthesis is equivalent to release, because they are not stored. Histamine, on the other hand, already exists but is in an inactive, bound state. When an appropriate stimulus occurs, such as an antigen-antibody interaction on a mast cell membrane, a chain of events is initiated that culminates in the exocytosis of the histamine-containing granules.

Regardless of the mechanism of activation, mediators can either be toxic (*e.g.*, complement–platelets) or nontoxic (*e.g.*, histamine–mast cell) to their cell of origin. In general, mediator release from the lung can be stimulated by immunologic, mechanical, chemical, and toxic factors. Specific examples of these factors and some of the mediators released are shown in Table 9–4.

Inflammatory Process

A principal role of mediators in the lung and elsewhere in the body is in the inflammatory reaction. As mentioned above, inflammation is a defensive reaction to injury that can be caused by various factors. One of the first responses that occurs is vasodilation. In the lung this is probably a result of the release of histamine from mast cells (located in the bronchi, around smaller blood vessels, in alveolar walls, and in the pleura) and of prostaglandins from endothelial cells. This is followed by swelling of the bronchial and vascular endothelium and by an increase in permeability. The altered endothelial wall promotes adherence of platelets and leukocytes and inflammatory cell infiltrates. The aggregation of platelets may initiate local coagulation, with fibrin deposition and thrombus formation. Released histamine can also produce airway smooth muscle contraction either by interaction with histamine receptors known as H_1 receptors, or indirectly by activation of subepithelial irritant receptors and reflex vagal activation.

The increased endothelial permeability that occurs leads to movement of fluid and protein from the vascular compartment into mucosal, interstitial, alveolar, or pleural regions, producing mucosal edema, pulmonary edema, and pleural effusion, respectively. The presence of increasing amounts of exudate can promote further destruction of ground substance and of other cells, with the release of additional mediators. Excess fluid and cells that accumulate are eventually drained from the region by lymph flow.

Inflammation is also accompanied by the chemotactive attraction of leukocytes. Polymorphonuclear neutrophils and then monocytes penetrate into the tissues and migrate to the damaged cells. Activation of leukocytes is believed to mediate the generalized Schwartzman reaction (microthrombi formation in small pulmonary vessels) that occurs in gram-negative endotoxemia. The mechanism appears to involve an increase in leukocyte thromboplastic activity, which triggers intravascular clotting. There are probably several humoral factors involved in the chemotaxis of leukocytes, including components of the complement system and prostaglandins.

The classic complement system is composed of 11 distinct serum proteins that, when activated, produce an amplification of tissue injury. Activation ocurrs through antibody interaction with the C1 trimolecular complex of complement, yielding various biologically active products with anaphylatoxic (C3a, C5a) and chemotactic (C5a, C5a des arg) properties. It has been postulated that, if the complement cascade is activated within the lung parenchyma as a result of pulmonary injury, neutrophils will accumulate and injure endothelial cells by generating hydrogen peroxide, superoxide anion, and other free radicals.

Cells at the site of injury that are damaged beyond their ability to self-repair undergo degeneration and autolysis via their lysosomal enzymes. Cellular debris created by this procedure is removed by phagocytosis by invading macrophages. If sufficient progenitor cells remain they will proliferate, and the progeny will migrate to the injured region to undergo differentiation and promote tissue reorganization (blood and lymphatic vessels, nerve connections). If a paucity of stem cells remain, fibroblasts will become activated to produce fibrotic tissue (scar).

FIBROSIS

The fibrogenic response serves to replace dead tissue and to entrap foreign particles. It is the final step in the inflammatory reaction, and occurs when "first-line" pulmonary defenses such as cough, phagocytosis by macrophage, and clearance by the mucociliary apparatus have failed. In most organs fibrosis is well tolerated and is beneficial to tissue healing and repair. However, in the lung, the production of a relatively small amount of fibrous tissue can be accompanied by considerable impairment of pulmonary function. Thus, the fibrotic process is particularly important to a study of the lung. The development of fibrosis in the lung is not a single process, but is a final common pathway of many biologic responses to numerous insulting agents. Important aspects of this response will be presented in the following discussion.

Collagen Biochemistry

The connective tissue of the lung normally helps to maintain the integrity and function of the organ. It is composed of collagen (60 to 70%), elastic fibers (25 to 35%), and proteoglycan (5%). In most species, the amount of each lung connective tissue component remains constant once adulthood is reached, with synthesis balancing degradation. However, if fibroblasts become activated, then additional collagen synthesis will occur, and fibrotic connective tissue will be deposited. Fibrotic lung disease is primarily a parenchymal disorder affecting alveolar types I and II, endothelial, and mesenchymal cells.

Collagen is the most abundant protein in the adult mammalian lung, and is probably the best characterized component of normal and fibrotic pulmonary tissue. Each collagen molecule is composed of three polypeptide chains (α), containing approximately 1100 amino acids coiled around each other in a triple helix. The polypeptide sequence is (x-y-glycine), in which x and y are usually proline-hydroxyproline and lysine-hydroxylysine. Following secretion collagen molecules aggregate into fibrils, which are stabilized by covalent cross-linkage between lysine and hydroxylysine residues. These covalent cross-links contribute to the insolubility and tensile characteristics of the molecule.

Five different types of collagen species have been identified in the lung, which vary in their amino acid sequence and in the types of polypeptide chains making up the triple helix. Type I collagen is the most abundant (60%) and widely distributed collagen in the lung. It can be found in bronchi, blood vessels, and interstitium, is composed of two α_1 (I) subtype chains and one α_2 subtype chain, and is formed in fibroblast and in type I epithelial cells.

Type II collagen has not been widely studied, but appears to be identical to collagen found in cartilage. It is composed of three α_1 (II) chains and is produced by chondrocytes in cartilaginous tissue of trachea and bronchi. Type III collagen is made up of three α_1 (III) chains, is generally widely distributed within the lung interstitium, and comprises about 30% of total collagen. Type III collagen is formed in fibroblasts and type I epithelial cells, and differs from collagen types I and II in that it contains disulfide cross links. Collagen types IV and V are found in basement membrane, and are the products of epithelial and endothelial cell synthesis.

Connective Tissue Accumulation

In certain chronic disorders connective tissue can accumulate in the lungs; these disorders are referred to as "fibrotic lung diseases," and can either be idiopathic or chemically induced. Over 150 environmental agents have been identified that are associated with lung fibrosis. The following is a brief (random) list of some known chemical factors: Bleomycin, paraquat, radiation (x-ray), N-nitroso-N-methylarethane, inhaled organic dusts (*e.g.,* silica, asbestos, berylium), toxic gases (*e.g.,* ozone, excess oxygen, nitrogen dioxide), cigarette smoke, phorbol myristate, busulfan chlorambucil, methotrexate, cyclophosphamide, azathioprine, practolol, pindolol, gold. Some fibrosis-producing agents act directly, while others are mediated through effector cells.

Regardless of etiology, the amount, type, location, and form of different connective tissue components within the lung become altered. For example, under normal conditions, the ratio of type I and type III collagen in the lung is approximately 2:1. However, in the presence of fibrosis, the ratio increases to 4:1. The accumulation of high tensile strength type I collagen in pulmonary fibrosis is consistent with the decreased lung compliance that occurs in this disorder.

The pulmonary fibrosis produced by some drugs (*e.g.,* bleomycin) can actually develop into the therapy-limiting factor. Chronic treatment with bleomycin to the extent that an accumulated total dose in excess of approximately 400 to 450 mg is reached is routinely associated with an incidence of pulmonary fibrosis of 10% and with a mortality rate of 1%. Patients who have had prior radiation exposure and those over 70 years of age are predisposed to pulmonary toxicity from bleomycin. Careful monitoring of bleomycin-treated patients is essential, therefore, because well-developed fibrosis is irreversible at this time.

Because of the importance of fibrotic lung disease as a clinical entity, considerable effort is being directed at understanding the factors that regulate collagen synthesis in the lung. Approximately 20 different animal models of pulmonary fibrosis have thus been developed. It is now known that, although collagen clearly accumulates in the scarred lung, it is often difficult to demonstrate the effect in animal studies on a concentration basis, because injury produces a corresponding elevation in parenchymal noncollagenous protein in the form of lymphocytes, macrophages, and vascular protein. It has also become apparent from studies of animal models of lung fibrosis that the localization of the deposited collagen is, in fact, the crucial point.

PULMONARY EDEMA

Increased Endothelium Permeability

Four mechanisms are generally thought to induce edema formation: elevated microvascular hydrostatic pressure; increased capillary permeability; obstruction to lymphatic drainage; and low vascular oncotic pressure. The first two mechanisms are believed to play the principal role within the lung. Pulmonary edema is classified into hydrostatic (cardiogenic, high-pressure) and permeability (noncardiogenic, low-pressure) forms, which can become manifested as either interstitial or alveolar edema (the latter form is generally an extension of interstitial edema).

Pulmonary edema is a common and important feature of many diseases of the lung. Inhalation of noxious gases and certain types of chemical and toxic injuries can cause massive pulmonary edema. Pulmonary edema has been reported as a result of exposure to phosgene, chlorine, the oxides of nitrogen and sulfur, ozone, metallic oxides, and acid fumes. With the exception of lymphatic obstruction, all types of pulmonary edema are caused by an elevated rate of fluid leakage from small vessels into the interstitial tissues of the lung. This can occur as a result of elevated hydrostatic pressure or of increased permeability of the endothelium.

The usual sequence of events in pulmonary edema following injury are as follows. There is first compensatory increase in lymph flow to drain the parenchyma and if the degree of injury is not too severe, this may be sufficient. However, if the lymph channels become engorged, corresponding pressure will be exerted on adjacent small airways, producing varying degrees of obstruction. If transudation is so extensive that lymph capacity is exceeded, alveolar wall edema will occur, leading to decreased compliance and to tachypnea. One method of studying the permeability of pulmonary capillaries is by measuring the lung lymph:plasma ratios of proteins of varying molecular weights.

The development of edema of the permeability type is always associated with alterations in the ultrastructural appearance of small blood vessels. These changes do not have to be of a great magnitude to be significant. Relatively small, localized lesions in the pulmonary endothelium are quite able to produce significant edema. Administration of the pulmonary edemagenic agent α-napthylthiourea to rats is known to produce edema after 1 hour, reaching a maximum by 3 to 4 hours postexposure. During this period of edema formation, electron photomicroscopy of the lung reveals the presence of intercellular gaps in the endothelium of pulmonary capillaries and vessels. These gaps can remain patent for several hours, and are similar to those seen during inflammation. Regeneration changes occur within 24 to 48 hours.

A relatively serious source of pulmonary edema is that associated with the use of narcotics, and can occur with both medical and illicit use. It has been described with heroin, morphine, methadone, propoxyphene, and ethchlorvynol. However, narcotic pulmonary edema is most commonly associated with heroin use by addicts. The mechanism of action is unknown, but can occur in some users within seconds; however, in most subjects, respiratory distress does not occur for some interval. Functional abnormalities can last for several weeks.

The vascular changes responsible for pulmonary edema formation can be the result of direct injury to the endothelial cell by the toxin or by the release of mediators. In the latter context, it is interesting to note that histamine-like permeability factors may cause leakage from bronchial venules, but they are not considered able to produce edema of pulmonary interstitial tissues or of alveoli. Possible candidates for the mediator in the parenchymal area are the prostaglandins, which are known to be potent local humoral agents.

Under normal circumstances, there are five principal mechanisms that protect the lung against edema: the lymphatic drainage system; low endothelial permeability to water; very low endothelial permeability to protein; plasma protein concentration; and perimicrovascular liquid pressure. Experiments with isolated rat alveolar epithelial cells suggest that these cells may also play a significant role in transporting fluid and, therefore, in resolving pulmonary edema. The mechanism appears to involve the active extrusion of sodium chloride, which carries an osmotic equivalent of water. The extent to which this process can be impaired by injury or enhanced by pharmacologic agents remains to be determined.

The aims of treatment for pulmonary edema are twofold: the maintenance of systemic arterial oxygenation, and a decrease in the sum of pressures that cause liquid filtration. Positive pressure breathing serves to inflate low-volume alveoli and to improve lung mechanics, resulting in fluid being driven from the airways. Hydrostatic fluid can be reduced in congestive heart failure by the administration of diuretics. An increase in water loss from the kidneys will decrease blood volume and total body water, with the lungs contributing their share.

Neurogenic Pulmonary Edema

Neurogenic pulmonary edema that occurs following acute injury to the central nervous system is believed to be the result of constriction of postcapillary arterioles in the lung by sympathetic nerve activation. A consequence of this hemodynamic change is a buildup of intraluminal pressure in the capillaries, and this increase in hydrostatic pressure creates a pressure-dependent leakage. There is some controversy as to whether this leakage is the result of "pore stretching" or represents an exaggeration of the normal exchange process. In general, the study of different experimental models shows that hydrostatic-type edema may develop without any detectable change in the ultrastructure of the pulmonary microvascular endothelium.

Pulmonary edema in patients without heart disease has been reported following propranolol administration when given to patients with pheochromocytoma. Administration of this β_1 and β_2 blocker is believed to leave α effects unopposed, resulting in arterial hypertension and in increased afterload. It has been suggested that it might be more reasonable to use a cardioselective β_1 blocker such as metoprolol tartrate rather than a nonselective β blocker such as propranolol.

SELECTED REFERENCES

Ahmed, T., et al.: Abnormal mucociliary transport in allergic patients with antigen-induced bronchospasm: Role of slow reacting substance of anaphylaxis. Am. Rev. Res. Dis., 124:110, 1981.

Cosio, M. G., Hale, K. A., and Newoehner, D. E.: Morphologic and morphometric effects of prolonged cigarette smoking on the small airways. Am. Rev. Resp. Dis., 122:265, 1980.

Evans, M. J.: Cell death and cell removal in small airways and alveoli. *In* Witschi, H., and Nettesheim, P. (eds.): Mechanisms in Respiratory Toxicology, Vol. 1, Boca Raton, CRC Press, 1982, pp. 189–218.

Evans, M. J., Stephens, R. J., and Freeman, G.: Renewal of pulmonary epithelium following oxidant injury. *In* Bocchuys, A. (eds.): Lung Cells in Disease, New York, North Holland, 1976, pp. 165–176.

Fulmer, J. D., and Crystal, R. G.: The biochemical basis of pulmonary function. *In* Crystal, R. G. (ed.): Lung Biology in Health and Disease, Vol. 2, New York, Marcel Dekker, 1976, pp. 419–466.

Gee, J. B. L., and Khandwala, A. S.: Motility, transport and endocytosis in lung defense cells. *In* Brain, J. D., Proctor, D. F., and Reid, L. M. (eds.): Respiratory Defense Mechanisms, Part II, New York, Marcel Dekker, 1977, pp. 926–981.

Hance, A. J., and Crystal, R. G.: Collagen. *In* Crystal, R. G. (ed.): Lung Biology in Health and Disease, Vol. 2, New York, Marcel Dekker, 1976, pp. 215–271.

Irivani, J., and Melville, G. N.: Mucociliary function in the respiratory tract as influenced by physicochemical factors. *In* Widdicombe, J. (ed.): Respiratory Pharmacology, Oxford, Pergamon Press, 1981, pp. 477–500.

Jeffery, P. K., and Reid, L.: The respiratory mucous membrane. *In* Brain, J., Proctor, D. F., and Reid, L. (eds.): Respiratory Defense Mechanisms, New York, Marcel Dekker, 1977, pp. 193–245.

Minty, B. D., Jordan, O., and Jones, J. G.: Rapid improvement in abnormal pulmonary epithelial permeability after stopping cigarettes. Br Med. J., 282:1183, 1981.

Nadel, J. A.: Autonomic regulation of airway submucosal gland secretion. *In* Hargreave, F. E. (ed.): Airway Reactivity: Mechanisms and Clinical Relevance, Toronto, Astra Pharmaceuticals, 1980, pp. 54–58.

Phipps, R. J.: The airway mucociliary system. Int. Rev. Physiol., 23:213, 1981.

Rennard, S., et al.: Lung connective tissue. *In* Witschi, H., and Nettesheim, P. (eds.): Mechanisms in Respiratory Toxicology, Vol. 2, Boca Raton, CRC Press, 1982, pp. 115–153.

10

External Toxins

ENVIRONMENTAL POLLUTANTS

Throughout our lives, we are exposed to an unending series of gaseous and particulate matter in our environment. Although most substances in the atmosphere to which we are exposed are relatively harmless, our lungs are in constant contact with large amounts of potentially harmful substances in the outdoor urban environment. It has been estimated that 100 million tons of particulates, mostly soot and dust, are spewed into the air yearly by such by-products of civilization as smoking chimneys, traffic, and farm and construction work. If all types of air pollution were eliminated, thousands of deaths per year might be prevented in the United States.

The reality of the danger of atmospheric pollutants on health in general and on the pulmonary system specifically is dramatized by the annual smog alerts in the Los Angeles basin, in which summer inversion layers trap increasing concentrations of pollutants. Within Los Angeles County, the maximum air pollution safety level, as determined by the Environmental Protection Agency (EPA), was exceeded more than 140 days in 1982. Over 4000 deaths have been attributed to three acute episodes of heavy air pollution alone (Meuse Valley, Belgium; Donara, Pennsylvania; and London).

The lung provides an easy port of entry for various undesirable agents, ranging from smog and industrial dusts to volatile agents such as glue used for psychological effects and chemical poisons. The death in 1984 of more than 2000 people in Bhopal, India, who breathed cyanide gas bears testimony to this fact. Because the lung presents the largest surface area that the body exposes to the environment, it merits the special attention of those concerned with the introduction of noxious factors into the body.

Ambient air pollution contributes toward both the occurrence and the aggravation of various types of pulmonary disorders. As mentioned above, air pollution may result from increased concentrations of gases or from airborne particulate matter. There are five major outdoor air pollutants that have been identified as accounting for 98% of our ambient air pollution. In descending order these are carbon monoxide, sulfur oxides, hydrocarbons, particulate matter (carbon), and nitrogen oxides. These materials find their way into the environment primarily through vehicular exhaust systems (90%), industry, electric power generation, space heating, and refuse disposal. In addition, photochemical oxidants dominate in areas in which automobiles produce most of the air pollution. The presence of all these factors in air jeopardizes human health, because the average adult at rest breathes in more than 500 cubic feet of air daily.

Carbon Monoxide

Carbon monoxide (CO) is the most common air pollutant in the United States, with more than 100 million tons emitted annually. Most CO comes from the incomplete combustion of organic materials by automobile engines, at a rate of about 2.4 pounds for each gallon of gasoline. Fortunately, CO does not appear to be accumulating in the atmosphere, apparently because soil bacteria can remove CO from the air above the soil and thus act as a CO sink. Depending on conditions, people can be exposed to CO concentrations ranging from 9 to 15 parts/million (ppm) at street level and up to 4000 ppm if they are fire fighters. A predictable and common cause of CO exposure is cigarette smoking.

The following are the major adverse effects of CO in normal people:

1. Decreased oxygen delivery: less oxygen bound to hemoglobin; increased affinity of remaining hemoglobin for oxygen, with decreased release at the tissue level; compensatory increase in red cell mass

2. Interference with oxygen binding to myoglobin and with cytochrome oxidase system

3. Reduced birth rate and increased neonatal mortality rate

4. Possible increase in atherosclerosis

These effects are best understood in relation to the interference of CO with oxygen (O_2) transport. Because CO has a several-hundredfold greater affinity for hemoglobin than does O_2, small amounts of CO result in relatively high concentrations of carboxyhemoglobin. For example, a person smoking one pack of cigarettes a day commonly has a five- to six-fold increase in carboxyhemoglobin level. In fact, smoking produces far higher CO tissue levels than almost any other environmental pollutant. This relative hypoxia can have a deleterious effect on highly respirable tissue, as in the developing fetus, in whom growth may be stunted. Patients with coronary artery or peripheral vascular disease are more prone to exercise-induced hypoxia at elevated CO levels because they are incapable of increasing their blood flow. Generally speaking, the lung itself shows very little morphologic damage from CO.

Sulfur Dioxide

Sulfur dioxide (SO_2), first described as a bronchoconstrictor agent in 1713, normally is almost absent from the environment. However, as the burning of fuels containing sulfur has increased, there has occurred a corresponding elevation in levels of SO_2 and of its oxidation product sulfur trioxide. Substantial irritation of mucous membranes of the upper respiratory tract occurs at levels of 10 to 25 ppm. Elderly patients with underlying bronchitis and emphysema are at particular risk, while asthmatics can be predicted to have increased bronchospasm. High levels of sulfur have also been associated with acute respiratory disease (*e.g.*, laryngotracheobronchitis) in otherwise unsymptomatic children and adults. SO_2 can also eventually form sulfuric acid, which appears to have a greater potency for irritation than does sulfur dioxide.

Nitrogen Dioxide

Nitrogen dioxide is produced by several manufacturing processes, including the production of almost all nitrogen-based explosives. However, as with CO, cigarette smoking produces higher tissue levels of nitrogen dioxide than almost any other environmental factor. Nitrogen dioxide primarily damages terminal airways and alveoli by forming nitric and nitrous acids. Toxic effects are variable, depending on level of exposure, duration of exposure, and sensitivity of the individual. Acute high levels of nitrogen dioxide produce pulmonary edema, while chronic exposure leads to bronchiolar fibrosis and to respiratory insufficiency.

Aerosols

In many situations, gases, heavy metals, and hydrocarbons can become dissolved or suspended in airborne particles (either as a liquid mist or a solid fume). Such particles are referred to as aerosols. The size of a particle that can physically exist as an aerosol ranges from approximately 0.01 to 50 μm in diameter. In practice, however, there is usually only concern with particles in the range of 0.5 to 25 μm. Those particles smaller than 0.5 μm tend to behave as a gas—that is, they are in constant, rapid, and random motion, and therefore, are not readily deposited. Those particles larger than 25 μm tend to settle out from the air by gravity. The major factors affecting particle deposition in the respiratory tract may be described as follows:

A. Physical Properties
　1. State: particle, mist, vapor, fumes, gas; adsorption of SO_2 onto particles or carbon, then carried into distal airways
　2. Size and density of particles, mist, or aerosol determine site of deposition
　3. Shape and permeability

    4. Solubility
       a. Particles
          (1) Insoluble (e.g., asbestos)—local action
          (2) Soluble (e.g., manganese compounds)—systematic effects
       b. Gases and vapors
          (1) Insoluble (e.g., oxides of nitrogen)—reach small air passages
          (2) Soluble (e.g., ammonia, SO_2)—reach nose and nasopharynx
    5. Hygroscopicity: increase in particle size while traveling down respiratory tract
    6. Electric charge: influences site of deposition
B. Chemical properties
    1. Acidity and alkalinity: toxic effect on cilia, cells, and enzyme systems
    2. Propensity to combine with substances in lung and tissues; local and systemic effects (e.g., CO, hydrogen cyanide, fluoride compounds)
    3. Fibrogenicity: asbestos and silica versus iron and carbon
    4. Antigenicity: stimulate antibodies (e.g., fungal spores, detergent enzymes)
C. Host factors: genetic, environmental, and acquired
    1. Lung defenses
       a. Genetic determinants: ciliary action, clearance rates (slow and rapid clearers), macrophage function
       b. Acquired determinants: agents influencing ciliary and macrophage function (e.g., drugs, cigarette smoke, temperature, alcohol)
    2. Anatomic and physiologic factors: breathing patterns, airways, (geometry).
    3. Immunologic state; allergic diathesis, atopy, tissue type

There are five principal mechanisms of aerosol deposition: electrostatic attraction; interception; impaction; sedimentation; and diffusion. The relative contribution of each depends on the particular droplet, and is subject to considerable mathematical modeling. In general, however, particles between 1 and 10 μm are deposited mainly through inertial impaction and sedimentation, while those smaller than 0.5 μm, if deposited at all, do so by diffusion.

The relative distribution of the deposited droplets depends on the aerodynamic properties of the particle (*e.g.*, shape, mass), water solubility, anatomy of the respiratory tract, and airflow characteristics. Information about these factors can be extremely useful in predicting the fate of inhaled aerosols. For example, from theoretic considerations and experimental studies, it has been determined that the mass median diameter of aerosol particles corresponds to certain sites of deposition (Fig. 10–1).

On the basis of these data, three generalizations may be made: the most dangerous particles—namely, those most prone to be deposited in the alveoli—range in size from 0.5 to 2.5 μm; deposition in the nasophar-yngeal region occurs primarily with larger particles, ranging from 2 to 50 μm; and only a small fraction of an aerosol becomes deposited in the tracheobronchial region. However, the portion that is deposited in this region tends to concentrate in areas of bifurcations and turbulent airflow, creating "hot spots." This pattern of deposition correlates with the frequency of cancer reported in that area. Therefore, both total deposition and regional distribution are important determinants of toxicity and therapeutic efficacy.

When a person breathes an aerosol cloud present in the environment, particles of varying size are taken in. Studies on their physical character-istics indicate that they exist in three major modes of particle size distribution. The smallest size (0.02 to 0.1 μm) is referred to as the nuclei mode. These particles are transient in nature, because they tend to coalesce into larger aggregates. They generally exist only in close proximity to their site of origin, such as major highways. When encountered, nuclei-mode particles may deposit in the pulmonary region if given the opportunity. However, at this small size, the particles will tend to act as gases and can be expired before deposition.

The next largest category is the fine mode (0.2 to 0.6 μm). Because of their size, these particles will deposit primarily in the pulmonary region, with an efficiency of 20 to 40%. The major fraction of particle mass in the fine mode is the result of combustive processes associated with fossil fuel power plants, vehicular exhaust industrial processes, domestic heating, hydrocarbon emissions from refineries, and fuel transportation. This group is composed of gases (SO_2, sulfur trioxide—SO_3, and nitrogen oxides), heavy metals (lead, manganese, vanadium), soot (graphite car-

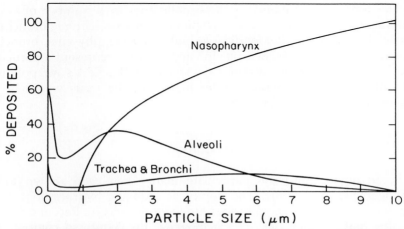

Figure 10–1. Relationship of particle size (mass median diameter) to depo-sition sites in the respiratory system.

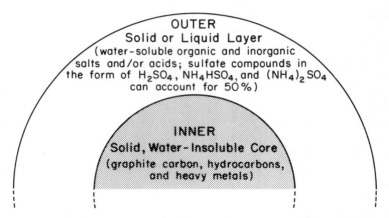

Figure 10–2. Cross section of a theoretic fine-mode aerosol particle.

bon), and assorted hydrocarbons. A present view of the structure of fine-mode particles is shown in Figure 10–2.

The largest aerosol particles are referred to as the coarse mode, and have a volume (mean size) of 5 to 10 μm. These particles originate in the atmosphere from man-made and natural sources. Natural sources include sand, soil, sea salt, and pollen. Components from human activities include silicates, aluminum, magnesium, and iron, which become airborne during mining, manufacturing, and agricultural processes. These particles are less homogeneous chemically than those in the fine mode, and are about twice as dense. Because of their size, coarse-mode particles will deposit primarily in the nasopharyngeal region, with an efficiency of 50 to 100%. Particles larger than 25 μm tend to settle to the ground because of their gravimetric mass.

The lung may respond to these pollutants in a number of ways, including acute nonspecific upper respiratory disease, chronic bronchitis, chronic obstructve ventilatory disease, pulmonary emphysema, bronchial asthma, and lung cancer. Because inhaled particles represent a particular threat to the respiratory system, a revision of the EPA's air pollution standard has been proposed. Under that plan, the focus would be on particles smaller than 10 μm.

Hydrocarbons

Some organic airborne particulate matter has been shown to be carcinogenic or mutagenic. The polycyclic aromatic hydrocarbons (*e.g.*, benzo[*a*]pyrene) have generally been the focus of concern. Recent evidence indicates that another class of carcinogens, the *N*-nitroso compounds, may be of equal significance. Assay of New York City air has shown that its molar *N*-nitroso concentration is equivalent to that of the polycyclic aromatic hydrocarbons in respirable 3.5-μm particles. In view of the fact that several hundred *N*-nitroso compounds have been found to be carcinogenic, obvious implications are raised.

Photochemical Oxidants

When heavy automobile use occurs during periods of stable atmospheric conditions, oxidizing air pollutants are formed with the aid of photochemical energy from the sun. Ozone and peroxyacetyl nitrate (PAN) are the major oxidants formed from automobile combustion. Eye irritation is the primary toxic effect of PAN, while ozone produces dryness of the mucosal membrane of the respiratory tract, headache, cough, bronchitis, and pulmonary edema in high concentrations. However, the exact effect of photochemical products on the health of those exposed to them is unknown.

Lead

The presence of lead in 45% of the gasoline sold is considered by the EPA to be a major public health concern. It has been estimated that there would have been 80% fewer cases of lead toxicity among children if there had been no lead in gasoline between 1977 and 1981. Pollution from leaded gas is believed to have contributed approximately 20% of the lead found in the blood of children with high lead concentrations. The toxic alert level is 25 µg/dl of blood. Legislation is now being considered to remove leaded gasoline from the marketplace.

OCCUPATIONAL HAZARDS

Inhalation is the principal route of workers' exposure to toxic substances. Occupational lung diseases, especially those resulting from mineral dusts, have been recognized for thousands of years. Today, industrial exposure of workers involves an ever-increasing number of chemically diverse agents, which can produce varying degrees of lung injury. All the industrial toxicants that produce lung disease through inhalation will not be discussed in this section. Instead, representative examples of different categories have been chosen, generally on the basis of the number of American workers exposed and on the type of pulmonary injury produced.

Irritants

Two types of lung toxins that affect millions of workers yearly are irritants and those that produce severe cell damage. Irritants are materials that inflame mucous surfaces. With few exceptions, the aqueous solubility of an irritant is the most important single factor determining its site of action within the respiratory tract. Highly soluble irritant gases (*e.g.*, ammonia, chlorine, SO_2) primarily affect the upper respiratory tract, and are usually free of systemic toxicity. Over 500,000 workers are exposed to ammonia and chlorine alone, which are primarily used in the fertilizer and chemical industries. Because these gases are water-soluble, they tend to be hydrated, and exposure usually results in upper airway removal and concentration. The result is bronchoconstriction resulting either from the direct effect of locally released mediators or from irritant reflexes (see Chap. 1), or from both. Edema and dyspnea often follow.

Compounds of intermediate solubility affect both upper respiratory tract and pulmonary tissue (*e.g.*, halogens, ozone, toluene diisocyanate). Insoluble materials such as NO_2 and phosgene produce severe respiratory damage with little or no upper airway irritation, and thus may be even more dangerous. These insoluble gases may have latency periods of up to 24 hours before the onset of symptoms.

An example of a nongaseous irritant is arsenic, which is used in the production of pesticides and pigments. About 1.5 million workers are exposed. Like ammonia and chlorine, arsenic produces a direct irritation of the nasopharyngeal and tracheobronchial regions. Bronchitis is the usual symptom, although inflammation of the larynx may also occur after chronic exposure.

An interesting historical note regarding arsenic involves Napoleon. It has been postulated that one factor contributing to his general decline in health while on St. Helena was chronic exposure to low levels of arsenic. At that time, arsenic was used for paint and pigments used in wallpaper. Under normal circumstances the arsenic is tightly bound. However, if moisture allows mold to grow, the enzymatic activity of these microbes can release volatile arsenic.

Cell Death

A number of inhaled chemicals can cause frank cell death as well as an inflammatory response to irritation (*e.g.*, ozone, NO_2, and phosgene). These gases are characterized by the important property of having low water solubility, which allows them to reach the more distal sites of the respiratory system, including the bronchioles and alveoli. Another important aspect of phosgene's action is the formation of hydrochloric acid (HCl) in the upper respiratory tract which inhibits its absorption so that the gas can penetrate further. Because epithelial type I cells are quite sensitive to toxins, they are a common locus of destruction. Organic solvents such as perchloroethylene (used in dry cleaning and metal degreasing) and xylene (used in manufacturing and as a general solvent) have a good chance to reach the lower levels of the lung, because they are also water-insoluble and quite volatile.

Chemicals inhaled through the lungs can also have significant effects on the body other than directly on the respiratory system. In the late 1970s, for example, male workers exposed to the soil fumigant 1,2-dibromo-3-chloropropane (used for plant nematodes) were reported to have low sperm counts, testicular atrophy, and lowered fertility as a result of chronic breathing of the chemical.

A recent study of hospital workers exposed to less than 50 ppm of ethylene oxide (used to sterilize supplies) for 6 months showed an increased frequency of sister chromatid exchanges in peripheral lymphocytes. This type of response is used to measure the chromosomal effects of mutagenic and carcinogenic agents. Although an accurate and safe exposure limit is difficult to determine for any chemical, this type of study raises serious concern about the accuracy of present safety standards, such as 50 ppm for ethylene oxide.

Fine particle deposition can also lead to cell death in the respiratory system. Cadmium oxide, which is used in welding, smelting, and electrical equipment manufacturing, for example, can penetrate alveoli. There the cadmium oxide causes interstitial edema with epithelial cell damage, leading to alveolar degeneration and development of emphysema.

Allergens

In addition to toxicants that can either irritate the respiratory tract directly or can damage the cells lining the airways, certain materials can produce disease indirectly by eliciting an allergic response. This mechanism involves the presence of circulating or fixed antibodies that are specific for the antigenic determinants of the inhaled material. When antigen and antibody interact, local allergic inflammations occur. Some materials that can produce chronic allergic alveolitis and inhalation disease are listed in Table 10–1. In addition, microbes present in sawdust from various types of wood, grains, and cheese, as well as in cork dust and bird droppings, are antigenic.

Pulmonary Fibrosis

One of the most diabolic forms of occupational lung disease is pulmonary fibrosis. Years of exposure to apparently innocuous material can produce ever so gradual decrements in pulmonary function, resulting eventually in a terribly debilitating and irreversible disease. Although pulmonary fibrosis was one of the earliest forms of occupational disease recognized, its incidence in the United States actually appears to be

Table 10–1. Examples of Inhalation Diseases*

Diseases	Agents	Occupation or Source of Exposure
Inorganic Dusts		
Silicosis	Silica	Minor, foundry worker, boiler scaler, sandblaster
Coal workers' pneumoconiosis (anthracosis)	Coal dust	Coal miner
Asbestosis	Asbestos	Asbestos miner or miller, insulation worker
Talcosis	Talc	Talc miner or miller, tire manufacturer, soapstone worker
Berylliosis	Beryllium	Beryllium extractor or manufacturer
Shaver's disease	Bauxite	Aluminum smelter
Organic Dusts		
Farmer's lung	*Micropolyspora faeni, Thermoactinomyces vulgaris*	Farmer working with moldy hay
Bagassosis	*Thermoactinomyces sacchari*	Sugarcane worker
Bird fancier's	Bird droppings and feathers	Pigeon breeder, bird owner
Humidifier lung	*Micropolyspora faeni, Thermoactinomyces vulgaris*	Occupant of building with humidifier in ventilation system
Mushroom worker's lung	Thermophilic actinomycetes	Mushroom composter
Sequoiosis	Thermophilic actinomycetes	Sawmill worker (redwood)
Maple bark stripper's disease	*Cryptostroma corticale*	Sawmill worker (maple)
Cheesewasher's disease	*Penicillin casei*	Cheese production worker
Pituitary snuff taker's lung	Pituitary powder	Patient with diabetes insipidus
Byssinosis	Cotton dust	Textile worker (cardroom worker)
Gases and Fumes		
Silo filler's disease	Oxides of nitrogen	Farmer
Occupational asthma	Toluene diisocyanate	Polyurethane foam worker

*(From Epstein, P. E.: Inhalation diseases. *In* Gong, H., and Drage, C. (eds.): The Respiratory System—A Core Curriculum, East Norwalk, Appleton-Century-Crofts, 1982, p. 298.

increasing. Some of the more prevalent inhalational sources of occupational pulmonary fibrosis are presented in Table 10–2.

Perhaps the most pervasive and best studied of these fibrotic agents is the group of hydrated silicates known as asbestos. This fibrous material varies in its chemical composition depending on the geochemistry of the area in which it is found. The most prevalent form is chrysolite $(3MgO \cdot 2SiO_2 \cdot 2H_2O)$, which is a serpentine asbestos that accounts for nearly 95% of the asbestos used worldwide.

Asbestos has been used for over 100 years. As early as 1918, health hazards relating to breathing asbestos were understood. Nevertheless, the technologic applications of asbestos are increasing worldwide, because asbestos material occurs in virtually all commercial minerals. It is estimated that 25 million Americans are exposed to asbestos yearly.

One of the more interesting contemporary aspects of asbestosis is the question of liability. Manville Corporation, the major American manufacturer, filed for reorganization under Chapter 11 of the United States Bankruptcy Code on August 26, 1982. This was deemed necessary not because of poor sales, but because of the thousands of lawsuits filed claiming health damage from exposure to asbestos products manufactured by Manville, and in anticipation of more suits. These claims are to a large degree from workers employed in the shipbuilding industry during World War II. It is the company's position that the federal government should share the responsibility.

The main problem with asbestos occurs if the fibers reach the interstitium, which they appear to be able to do if the particle size is 5×0.3 μm. Filamentous particles in the range of 30 to 60 μm can also reach the alveoli because long narrow particles have a low settling velocity. In fact, longer fibers have been associated with greater toxicity. In such a situation, the lung has no effective mechanisms either to degrade or remove the material, as might be found at higher levels of the respiratory pathway. Therefore, asbestos fibers that reach the interstitium have a tendency just to remain there and form fibrous deposits. The body does, however, try to remove the material by mobilizing macrophages. Unfortunately, this generally proves ineffective and, in fact, may be deleterious.

One theory of asbestos-induced pulmonary fibrosis suggests that, when pulmonary macrophages ingest the asbestos particles, they are forced to release lysosomal enzymes, which cause autolytic destruction of the macrophages and adjacent cell injury. In addition, phospholipids released concurrently are believed to stimulate fibroblasts in the area to increase synthesis, release, and deposition of collagen. Because the silica particles are not digested, they are eventually released intact back into interstitial cells, in which they are once again free to begin the cycle.

More recent evidence, based on the interaction of asbestos with erythrocyte membranes, suggests that intracellular lysosomal rupture may be unrelated to the cell deaths caused by asbestos in the lung. These studies indicate an interaction between positive charges on the asbestos

Table 10–2. Principal Industrial Toxicants Producing Pulmonary Fibrosis Through Inhalation

Toxicant	Chemical Composition
Aluminum dust	Aluminum and small amount of Al_2O_3
Aluminum	Al_2O_3
Tungsten, titanium, and tantalum carbides	
Coal dust	Coal plus SiO_2 and other minerals
Iron oxides	Fe_2O_3
Kaolin	$Al_4Si_4O_{10}$ (OH)$_8$ plus crystalline SiO_2
Silica	SiO_2
Talc	$Mg_6(Si)_2)OH_4$

fiber surface and negatively charged sialic acid residues on the plasma membrane, leading to a disruption of the normal permeability barrier to ions. The result is a loss of ion homeostasis (*e.g.*, calcium, sodium) followed by cell death. A more speculative additional alternative has been proposed involving the release of oxygen free radicals from macrophages and other inflammatory cells.

As mentioned above, there can occur an extremely long exposure period to asbestos before significant pulmonary toxicity can be documented. American shipworkers during World War II, for example, had latent periods of several decades before some of their problems became apparent. Clearly, the length of time before clinical symptoms become apparent depends on several factors, including intensity and duration of exposure and the presence of potentiating factors such as cigarette smoking or other pneumotoxins.

Occupational exposure to a pulmonary toxin is not the only way in which pulmonary fibrosis can occur. More benign opportunities also appear to exist. Since 1956, for example, there have been 43 cases of diffuse interstitial pulmonary disease attributed to hair spray inhalation. Exposure is characterized by frequent daily use for many years. The exact causative substance is unknown, although a lacquering agent (copolymer of maleic anhydride and butyric alcohol) has been detected in human lung biopsy samples. In infants and small children, the accidental inhalation of large amounts of talcum powder may lead to acute diffuse or fatal pneumonia. Zirconium has been removed from aerosol antiperspirants by the FDA because of its association with the formation of lung nodules.

Cancer

Of the various types of toxic responses that the lung can have, cancer is undoubtedly the most life-threatening. It is all the more ironic, then, that the principal source of lung cancer is voluntary exposure to cigarette smoke. Numerous studies have dealt with the carcinogenicity of cigarette smoke components and the epidemiology of smoking and lung cancer, so these subjects will not be covered here.

In addition to cigarette smoking, several substances are also associated with malignant transformations in the human lung (Table 10–3). Inhalation of carcinogenic material should not be viewed, however, as an exclusive threat to the lung. Occupational exposure to volatile agents such as anilines and benzene has also been shown to be associated with cancer of the bladder and leukemia, respectively.

Recent epidemiologic evidence indicates that asbestos is a causal factor for human mesothelioma (peritoneal, pericardial, pleural) and lung cancer. The risk of tumor development appears to be influenced by the fiber type and by personal habits such as smoking. The latent period for tumor development following occupational exposure usually exceeds 20 years, with a marked increase in risk after 30 to 35 years. An increased risk of mesothelioma has also been reported for persons residing near industrial sources of asbestos and for spouses and pets of workers in asbestos-related occupations.

Concern has also been expressed over airborne asbestos fibers causing cancer deaths in the general public. A National Research Council committee has estimated that approximately nine deaths/million will occur due to mesothelioma. The figure is based on 400 fibers/m^3 being breathed throughout life.

DRUGS OF ABUSE

Tobacco

In addition to serving as a window of access for toxicants and therapeutic agents, the respiratory system has also been used for centuries as a route for the self-administration of psychoactive agents. The most widely used drug in this regard is, of course, tobacco. The derivation of the word may, in fact, come from that for a two-pronged tube used by natives to take snuff. The major interest in tobacco during its early days was medical. It was introduced into Europe in the late 16th century as an herb for the treatment of disorders ranging from flatulence to labor pains. Its merit was debated over the next several centuries, resulting in nicotine being dropped from the United States Pharmacopeia in the 1890s.

As its medicinal use declined, however, there was a corresponding increase in its recreational use. Tobacco was not only smoked but also taken as snuff—Napoleon is said to have used 7 pounds of snuff a month. In the United States, the transition to smoking as the principal method of tobacco use occurred during the first quarter of the 20th century.

The adverse health effects of smoking are well known. The Public Health Service of the United States, in its 1979 report to Congress, stated that "Cigarette smoking is the single most important environmental factor contributing to premature mortality in the United States." The major

Table 10–3. Inhalation of Some Industrial Toxicants Associated with Lung Cancer

Toxicant	Site
Asbestos (Mg, Ca fibrous silicates)	Pulmonary parenchyma
Arsenic (As_2O_3, AsH_3, $Pb_3(AsO_4)_2$)	Upper airways (bronchioles, larynx)
Chromium (Na_2CrO_4 and other salts)	Nasopharynx and upper airways
Coke oven emissions (polycyclic hydro- carbons, oxides of sulfur and nitrogen)	Tracheobronchi
Halo ethers (bis-(chloromethyl)ether)	Upper respiratory tract
Radionuclides (uranium, radium, radon gas)	
Nickel (elemental as well as carbonyl, subsulfide, and oxide forms)	Nasal mucosa and bronchi

Table 10–4. Major Toxic Agents in Cigarette Smoke*

Gas Phase (90% of total)	Particulate Phase (less than 10% of total)
Carbon dioxide	Nicotine
Nitrosamines	"Tar" (*e.g.*, polycyclic aromatic
Hydrazine	hydrocarbons)
Vinyl chloride	Cresols
Urethane	Phenol
Formaldehyde	DDT
Hydrogen cynanide	Hydroquinone
Acrolein	Pyridine
Acetaldehyde	Endrin
Nitrogen oxides	Metals
Ammonia	Butylamine
Pyridine	Dimethylamine
Carbon monoxide	Furfural
Acrylonitrile	
Volatile sulfur-containing compounds	

*(Adapted from Smoking and Health: A Report of the Surgeon General, Washington, DC, U.S. Department of Health, Education, and Welfare, 1979.)

diseases related to chronic smoking include lung cancer, heart disease, bronchitis and emphysema, peptic ulcer, and complications of pregnancy and infant health.

The chemical composition of cigarette smoke is complex; over 2000 components have been identified. Some of the major toxic agents in cigarette smoke are shown in Table 10–4. Perhaps the most important, in terms of the cardiovascular system, is nicotine. Inhalation is a very effective drug delivery system for nicotine, with up to 90% being absorbed. In tobacco smoke aerosols, nicotine is primarily associated with particles ranging from 0.35 to 0.43 μm in aerodynamic diameter, from which transfer into the bloodstream occurs.

Nicotine causes the release of catecholamines from the adrenals and sympathetic nerve endings. This produces an elevation in heart rate and blood pressure, which increases the heart's need for oxygen. In cases of pre-existing impaired coronary blood flow, the risk of heart attack increases. Cigarette smoking is also linked with low levels of high-density lipoproteins (HDL), which are believed to provide endogenous protection against cholesterol accumulation in atherosclerosis. The risk of coronary heart disease decreases rapidly if smoking is stopped.

Studies from numerous countries demonstrate a clear increase in bronchitis and emphysema as a function of quantity and duration of smoking. The precise mechanism whereby cigarette smoke produces lung disease is unknown, but is undoubtedly multifactorial. Likely targets include alveolar surfactant, ciliated cells, and macrophages, and possibly effects on proteolytic enzymes, interference with immune mechanisms, and genetic predisposition.

One proposed explanation for the association between cigarette smoking and the development of emphysema *in humans* is an increase in the elastase burden of the lungs of smokers as a result of the presence of larger numbers of polymorphonuclear neutrophils and alveolar macrophages, inactivation of lung antielastases by oxidants in cigarette smoke, and, the correlation of nicotine content with inhibition of antielastase function. These factors would be particularly significant in individuals with inherited intermediate or severe alpha$_1$-antitrypsin (AAT) deficiency. Therefore, these independent but mutually reinforcing factors could lead to a net increase in the lung's protease activity in susceptible persons.

Lung cancer is the most common malignant cause of death in North America. The male death rate in 1980 was 70/100,000/year, and is clearly correlated with cigarette consumption. No specific cell type has been consistently linked to lung cancer. Current evidence also suggests an increased incidence of cancer in other parts of the respiratory system, such as the mouth, larynx, and esophagus. In addition, smokers have a higher rate of cancer of the urinary bladder, kidney, and pancreas. Noncancer-related pathology also occurs, of course, as a result of chronic smoking. For example, the incidence of peptic ulcers in smokers is about 1.7 times that of nonsmokers, and the mortality rate from peptic ulcer is about twice as high in smokers.

Maternal smoking during pregnancy is associated with decreased infant birth weight and increased incidence of prematurity, spontaneous abortion, stillbirth, and neonatal death. The exact underlying mechanisms are unknown. However, the higher levels of carboxyhemoglobin in smokers is believed to produce a state of relative hypoxia, thus interfering with normal development. In heavy smokers the carboxyhemoglobin level may rise to as high as 15%, and undoubtedly increases the risk of angina and possibly atherosclerotic plaque development.

Smoking may also contribute to the gender longevity gap. The results of a study published in 1983 support the conclusion that virtually all of the increase in the difference between male and female longevity since 1930 is attributable to the effects of cigarette smoking. Although this explanation is not universally accepted by experts in the field, smoking is undoubtedly a significant contributor to the longevity differential between men and women.

Cocaine

Coca leaves appear to have been used as long as 1500 years ago in Peru. Although generally chewed, the smoking of coca paste (60 to 80% cocaine sulfate) is also a popular pastime. The use of cocaine has increased in developed countries over the last decade. It was estimated that, in 1980, 40 metric tons of illegal cocaine entered the United States, and sold for an estimated 30 billion dollars.

Cocaine is commonly taken intranasally ("snorted") to avoid the use of a needle. The powder is usually arranged in 3- × 5-cm lines containing about 25 mg and inhaled through a straw. Its effects are usually described as euphoriant, and are similar to those produced by amphetamines. A dose of 25 mg intransally can produce a "high." In snorting, the objective is to get the cocaine hydrochloride as high as possible into the nasal passages so that it has access to the blood vessels of the nasal mucosa for absorption. Two side effects of this method of administration are damage to the septum (vasoconstriction) and a runny nose (rebound vasodilation).

In addition to snorting, a popular method of intake is by smoking. However, the hydrochloride salt, which is the usual street form of cocaine, is not satisfactory for this route of administration. The solution to this drug delivery problem has been to turn the cocaine hydrochloride into its free base. In addition to producing a substance more palatable for smoking, "free basing" is done to remove water-soluble adherants and to increase lipid solubility of the cocaine for better absorption. The "free basing" procedure is dangerous because it involves the use of volatile, explosive solvents, which have been known to cause serious injury to the amateur chemist. Once formed, however, cocaine free base can readily be smoked.

Illicit drug usage of other types can result in the formation of "filler" emboli in pulmonary capillaries. This occurs when compounds designed for oral use are injected intravenously. These oral preparations consist largely of fillers such as talc or starch, and this insoluble material accumulates in pulmonary capillaries to produce thrombosis, fibrosis, or pulmonary hypertension.

Marihuana

Marihuana is composed of various cannabinoids produced by several varieties of hemp plant. It is usually obtained from the flowering tops, which have a high concentration, although any part of the plant may be used. Basically, the material is cut, dried, chopped, and incorporated into cigarettes. Most psychological effects of marihuana are produced by Δ^9-tetrahydrocannabinol (THC), an isomer of tetrahydrocannabinol. THC is approximately three times more potent when smoked than when taken orally. In the United States, the THC content of marihuana ranges from 0.5 to 6%. Of this, no more than 50% is absorbed. Over 60% of young American adults have reported some experience with marihuana.

Marihuana smokers frequently report dry mouth and throat, which is probably the result of heat rather than of a constituent of the smoke. Chronic smoking of marihuana has been associated with nonspecific lung responses such as bronchitis and asthma. Adverse effects have also been noted on certain pulmonary function tests and on bronchial epithelial morphology. Interestingly, the acute effect of oral, intravenous, or aerosol

THC in the respiratory tract is bronchodilation. In humans, bronchodilation can be produced by 15 mg of THC orally or by smoking marihuana containing 2% of THC in amounts of 7 mg of marihuana/kg of body weight. The bronchodilator effect is not caused either by a decrease in vagal tone or by an increase in sympathetic activity, because neither atropine nor propranolol has any influence. Recent evidence suggests that the effect could be the result of THC stimulating lung phospholipase to produce prostaglandin E (PGE). The potency of THC as a bronchodilator is approximately 0.1% that of isoproterenol when tested on isolated tracheal smooth muscle. The potential clinical application of this effect of THC is being modestly investigated at the present time, as are other pharmacologic properties (*e.g.*, antiemesis, reduction of intraocular pressure in glaucoma). Of particular interest is whether or not this potentially beneficial bronchodilator effect can be separated from undesirable physiologic or psychological effects.

Volatile Agents

The intoxicating and euphorigenic effects of gases such as nitrous oxide and ethyl ether were actually recognized before their clinical application as anesthetics was discovered. Today, with the availability of a wide variety of volatile materials, inhalant abuse has become a popular alternative to abuse of less readily available and more expensive intoxicants.

The use of commercial solvents as a means of achieving an intoxicant state has a relatively short history. The origin of this practice has been ascribed to California during the late 1950s. Glue and gasoline sniffing are among the more popular forms of expression. Between 10 and 15% of young adults (18 to 25 years old) have indicated some experience with inhalants. In fact, a survey of senior high school students in 1980 indicated that inhalants were the fourth most prevalent form of drug use, following alcohol, cigarettes, and marihuana. Government figures indicate, however, that inhalant abusers are more likely to be involved with the criminal justice system, and at an earlier age.

The most immediate physical threat from inhalant abuse is death by suffocation or choking. One of the most popular methods of inhaling a volatile material is to accumulate a large volume in a plastic bag and to breathe from it. Because extremely high concentrations can be achieved in this manner, varying degrees of hypoxia or even death can occur. Unfortunately, inhalant abusers can be rather creative to this end. Nitrous oxide, for example, is routinely used as a propellant in aerosol dispensers for products such as whipped cream. A recent death from the inhalation abuse of this gas has raised the question of whether some type of regulation may be necessary for this apparently innocent and imaginative form of packaging.

The toxicity produced by inhaled material obviously depends on the substance in question, but is typically associated with respiratory problems. Inhalation of aerosol propellants containing fluorinated hydrocarbons, however, can produce cardiac toxicity, including arrhythmias and ischemia. Chlorinated solvents, such as trichlorethylene, can also depress myocardial contractility. Pulmonary hypertension is associated with ketone inhalation, while neurologic impairment may occur with various solvents, including lacquer thinner and aerosol paints. Deliberate sniffing of gasoline fumes has led to death. In Canada, the death of two adolescents has been attributed to inhalation of fumes from a commonly used typewriter correcting fluid, which contained the volatile solvent 1,1,1-trichloroethane.

Recent evidence also suggests that medical personnel exposed to gaseous anesthetics may suffer untoward toxicity. For example, nurse-anesthetists who work in the operating room while pregnant appear to have a higher risk of bearing an infant with a birth defect than either anesthetists who do not administer anesthesia during their pregnancy or women in the general population. This finding emerged from a survey of 695 births; of the 96 major and minor defects reported, 84% involved children who were born to mothers who administered anesthesia during their pregnancies.

Other studies have also suggested that the rate of spontaneous abortion in this population is two- to four-fold greater than that in the general public. Although not proving a cause-and-effect relationship, these findings strongly suggest that extreme caution should be exercised in exposing pregnant nurses to gaseous substances that can cross the placenta easily. The National Institute for Occupational Safety and Health has estimated that approximately 250,000 workers are exposed to anesthestia vapors each year.

Amyl Nitrite

Amyl nitrite is a highly volatile substance that has been used therapeutically since 1867 for the treatment of angina pectoris. The advent of other vasodilators such as nitroglycerin, however, precipitated a decline in its therapeutic value. It has been misused since at least 1930 as a recreational inhalant. It is available by prescription in glass vials that are "popped" or "snapped." An analog with similar pharmacologic effects, butyl nitrite, is legally available as a room deodorizer or as liquid incense. The fumes can either be inhaled directly from the bottle, or an inhaling device can be purchased with a wick that is dipped into the liquid. It is estimated that in 1979 over 250 million recreational doses of amyl and butyl nitrites were sold.

The principal pharmacologic effect of this substance is smooth muscle relaxation. One possible reason for its early and extensive use by male homosexuals was to produce relaxation of the anal sphincter muscle. The drug has also been inaccurately associated with an aphrodisiac effect, which probably explains why it is sniffed today by heterosexuals. Because some frequent users claim that they can no longer perform sexually without the use of nitrites, psychological dependence may be a possible side effect in selected individuals. Finally, it has been suggested that the use of amyl nitrite may depress the immune system and favor the development of Kaposi's sarcoma in male homosexuals.

HERBICIDES AND INSECTICIDES

Paraquat

Paraquat is a bipyridyl herbicide used in more than 130 countries. It is associated with serious lung disease primarily as a result of accidental or intentional ingestion of the liquid or, in an occupational setting, from percutaneus absorption of spray solution. The severity of lung injury depends on the dose and route of exposure. Intestinal absorption is the most severe, with 20 to 40 mg/kg of body weight probably being a fatal dose. Death usually results either from acute lung inflammation or from chronic lung fibrosis. However, renal and liver damage can also be significant. Because paraquat's destructive effects are believed to be the result of superoxide formation, oxygen therapy may potentiate the injury. Large doses of beclomethasone or prednisone have been recommended for drug therapy although gastric lavage, hemoperfusion, and other strategies have been used.

Exposure to diluted paraquat spray mist is not usually associated with systemic toxicity, because most inhaled droplets are too large (>200 μm in mean diameter) to reach the alveolar spaces, and are deposited in the mucosa of the upper respiratory tract. This results in local irritation leading to nosebleed, sore throat, and coughing. The current paraquat threshold limit value for respirable particles (<7 μm) is 100 μg/m^3.

Organophosphates

Organophosphates such as parathion and malathion can be absorbed through the skin, orally, or by inhalation. Their principal pharmacologic effect is the production of excess cholinergic activity by inhibition of acetylcholinesterase at nerve endings. The result is increased parasympathetic activity, including bronchial secretions and pulmonary edema. Farm workers exposed to sprayed crops and employees involved in their manufacture and transport are those primarily at risk. Treatment consists of antagonizing cholinergic activity with atropine and of reactivating the enzyme with pralidoxime.

Inhibition of respiratory tract acetylcholinesterase is also the mechanism of nerve agents such as soman, sarin, and tabun. The cause of death from these toxins is anoxia caused by sudden respiratory paralysis, severe bronchial constriction, excess accumulations of bronchial and salivary gland secretions, and weakness of the accessory muscles of respiration.

Insecticides such as pyrethrum and toxaphene have been associated with subacute extrinsic allergic "alveolitis" and bilateral pneumonic disease, respectively. Pyrethrum may represent a particular hazard because it is sometimes present in carbamate insectides that are sprayed.

INDOOR AIR POLLUTANTS

Recently, there has been an increase in concern over possible health hazards associated with contemporary airborne contaminants in the home and in other microenvironments. For example, a study done by the Oak Ridge National Laboratory found the level and variety of potentially harmful chemicals in the air of 40 suburban homes to be several times greater than that found outdoors. Government regulations are now being imposed to limit indoor exposure to sidestream tobacco smoke (from burning cigarettes), asbestos, formaldehyde, and radon. Indoor exposure and possible health consequences of other agents have not been adequately evaluated; these include NO_2 and CO, to which most exposure appears to be indoors. Although the medical impact of many indoor pollutants is largely speculative at this time, perhaps there are maladies that are primarily the result of or exacerbated by these factors. Major indoor pollutants and their sources are listed in Table 10-5.

Fuels

Our early cave-dwelling ancestors lived with contaminated air, as evidenced by the soot found on ceilings in prehistoric caves. Today, increased sales of wood- and coal-burning stoves and kerosene heaters indicate a return to "dirty" heating fuels. It is known that emissions from these heating sources contain toxic and carcinogenic particles and gas combustion by-products.

Elevated concentrations of NO_2 or CO have been reported in homes and schools in which kerosene heaters and unvented gas heaters are used. Numerous studies indicate NO_2 levels to be severalfold higher than the National Ambient Air Quality Standard ($100 \ \mu g/m^3$). Exposure to NO_2 can cause various pulmonary toxicologic effects, including pulmonary edema, bronchoconstriction, and increased infection rates. CO accumulation is a common cause of death among urban poor when a gas stove is used for heating. Individuals with angina pectoris appear to be extremely sensitive to as little as 1% carboxyhemoglobin in their blood.

Tobacco Smoke

There is increasing evidence that passive exposure to tobacco smoke may affect respiratory health. Cardiovascular, central nervous system, and respiratory changes have been reported in nonsmokers who are exposed to smoke. There have been consistent findings correlating parental cigarette consumption with respiratory symptoms and increased morbidity rates in children. For example, a recent longitudinal, well-controlled study suggests that passive exposure to maternal cigarette smoke may have important effects on the development of pulmonary function in children. In this study, it was found that, in children exposed to a mother

Table 10–5. Summary of Indoor Nonoccupational Pollutants*

Pollutant	Major Emission Sources
Origin: Predominantly Outdoors	
Sulfur oxides (gases, particles)	Fuel combustion, smelters
Ozone	Photochemical reactions
Pollens	Trees, grass, weeds, plants
Lead, manganese	Automobiles
Calcium, chlorine, silicon, cadmium	Suspension of soils, industrial emissions
Organic substances	Petrochemical solvents, natural sources, vaporization of unburned fuels
Origin: Indoors and Outdoors	
Nitric oxide, nitrogen dioxide	Fuel burning
Carbon monoxide	Fuel burning
Carbon dioxide	Metabolic activity, combustion
Particles	Resuspension, condensation of vapors, combustion products
Water vapor	Biologic activity, combustion, evaporation
Organic substances	Volatilization, combustion, paint, metabolic action, pesticides
Spores	Fungi, molds
Origin: Predominantly Indoors	
Radon	Building construction materials (concrete, stone), water
Formaldehyde	Particleboard, insulation, furnishings, tobacco smoke
Asbestos, mineral, and synthetic fibers	Fire retardant materials, insulation
Organic substances	Adhesives, solvents, cooking, cosmetics
Ammonia	Metabolic activity, cleaning products
Polycyclic hydrocarbons, arsenic, nicotine, acrolein, and so forth	Tobacco smoke
Mercury	Fungicides, paints, spills in dental care facilities or laboratories, thermometer breakage
Aerosols	Consumer products
Microorganisms	People, animals, plants
Allergens	House dust, animal dander, insect parts

*(From Spengler, J. D., and Sexton, K.: Indoor air pollution: A public health perspective. Science, 221:11, 1983. Copyright 1983 by the American Association for the Advancement of Science.)

who smoked, the expected increase in FEV_1 was decreased by 10.7, 9.5, and 7.0% after 1, 2, and 5 years, respectively. Some evidence also indicates an association between tobacco smoke exposure of nonsmoking wives and an increased rate of lung cancer.

Radon

Radon is a radioactive decay product of radium 226, which is normally found in building material made from earth-crusted components (rock, soil). Because it is a gas, radon can diffuse into indoor air from the ground or from building materials. Although radon gas itself gives a small radiation dose, it decays into two solid α-emitting, short-lived daughters; these are inhaled and deposited on the bronchial tree, and they deliver a dose that is carcinogenic.

Radon first emerged as a health issue during the 1950s, when uranium miners were found to have higher rates of lung cancer. Recently, concern about radon gas in homes has grown. In a 1984 study by the National Council on Radiation Protection and Measurements, a warning was issued in regard to the potential buildup of radon. Ironically, homes with superior insulation are most at risk, because there is less air exchange.

Some American homes have radon levels with a significant potential for causing deleterious health defects. As many as 10,000 deaths/year from lung cancer have been estimated to be the result of in-home exposure to radon. Because indigenous radium content varies according to region, exposure concentrations are geographically dependent.

Microorganisms and Allergens

Inhalation of biologic aerosols is a primary mechanism of contagion for many acute respiratory infections. Tuberculosis, measles, smallpox, and staphylococci are known to be transmitted by forced air ventilation systems in schools and hospitals. Legionnaires' disease (*Legionella pneumophila*) and humidifier fever are classic examples of air conditioning-related pathogen transfer. In April of 1983, the bone marrow transplant center at Roswell Park Memorial Institute in New York was closed because a fungus in the air system infected seven patients, four of whom died from aspergillosis.

Because high humidity favors the growth of mold and fungi, humid climates are more prone to this type of allergenic problem. More and more new buildings now feature reduced ventilation and increased use of untreated recirculated air. Such a reduction in fresh air may contribute to increased rates of infection and allergy. This potentially may be highly significant, because respiratory ailments account for the majority of acute conditions, with high medical costs and lost time from work or school.

Formaldehyde

Various types of building materials, as well as carpets and draperies and some types of foam insulation, contain formaldehyde. Over a period of several years (the half-life of its emission is 4.4 years), formaldehyde is released from these sources into the home atmosphere. Formaldehyde, therefore, is usually inhaled, although ingestion or topical contact may also produce adverse effects. The concern over formaldehyde in the last few years is a result of its mutagenic activity in microorganisms and its production of nasopharyngeal carcinoma in laboratory rodents. Human studies show eye irritation at levels of formaldehyde routinely found in homes worldwide. In addition, chronic inhalation of low levels (approximately 1 ppm) may be associated with subtle CNS changes. This level has been reported in several studies of mobile homes.

Asbestos Fibers

There is a large potential for public exposure to asbestos because of its widespread use. As mentioned previously, increases in incidence of lung cancers, pleural and peritoneal mesotheliomas, and gastrointestinal tract cancers have been linked to occupational exposure to asbestos. Risk to the general public in nonoccupational settings is, however, unknown. Particular concern has been focused on schools because of the potential exposure of children to deteriorating asbestos-containing material. Attempts to monitor airborne asbestos have proven difficult, because exposure is intermittent because of episodic disruptions of the material.

SELECTED REFERENCES

Boyd, J. T.: Climate, air pollution and mortality. Br. J. Prevent. Soc. Med., 14:123, 1960.

Brain, J. D., and Valberg, P. A.: Deposition of aerosol in the respiratory tract. Am. Rev. Resp. Dis. 120:1325, 1979.

Epstein, P.: Inhalation diseases. In Gong, H., and Drage, C. W. (eds.): The Respiratory System: A Core Curriculum, Norwalk, Appleton-Century-Crofts, 1980, pp. 297–310.

Farber, J. L.: How do mineral dusts cause lung injury? Lab. Invest., 49:379, 1983.

Kennedy, G., and Trochimowicz, H.: Inhalation toxicology. In Hayes, A. (ed.): Principles of Methods of Toxicology. Raven Press, New York, 1982, pp. 185–207.

Lippmann, M.: Regional deposition of particles in the human respiratory tract. In Lee, D. H. K., Falk, H. L., and Murphy, S. D. (eds.): Handbook of Physiology, Sec. 9: Reaction to Environmental Agents, Bethesda, MD, American Physiology Society, 1977, pp. 213–232.

Menzel, D. B., and McClellan, R. O.: Toxic responses of the respiratory system. In Doull, J., Klaasen, C., and Amdur, M. (eds.): Toxicology: The Basic Sciences of Poisons, 2nd edition, New York, Macmillan, 1980, pp. 246–274.

Morgan, W. K. G.: The effects of particles, vapors, fumes, and gases. Eur. J. Resp. Dis., 63(Suppl. 123):7, 1982.

Index

Note: Numbers in *italics* refer to illustrations; numbers followed by (t) indicate tables

189

Saunders Monographs In Pharmacology and Therapeutics

SAUNDERS MONOGRAPHS IN PHARMACOLOGY AND THERAPEUTICS (SMPT)—

A series of important monographs featuring highly-focused topics with an academic orientation. Unsurpassed in clarity and depth of coverage, each volume in the series offers state-of-the-art coverage of a specific issue or a recent advance in clinical therapeutics. Each superbly-illustrated title is written and edited by experts of widely-recognized ability and undisputed authority. In fact, SMPT's list of authors is a virtual "Who's Who" of pharmacologic therapeutics.

Join the SMPT Subscriber Plan. You'll receive each new volume in the series upon publication—one to three titles publish each year—and you'll save postage and handling costs! Or you may order SMPT titles individually. If not completely satisfied with any volume, you may return it with the invoice within 30 days at no further obligation.

Timely, in-depth coverage you can count on . . . Enroll in the Subscriber Plan for SAUNDERS MONOGRAPHS IN PHARMACOLOGY AND THERAPEUTICS today!

Available from your bookstore or the publisher.

Complete and Mail Today!

☑ YES! Enroll me in the SAUNDERS MONOGRAPHS IN PHARMACOLOGY AND THERAPEUTICS Subscriber Plan so that I may receive future titles in the series immediately upon publication, and save postage and handling costs! If not completely satisfied with any volume, I may return it with the invoice within 30 days at no further obligation.

Name _____

Address _____

City _____ State_____ ZIP_____

☐ Credit my
   salesman